ten keys that cure

Cure

bible truths for better health *today*

D1124897

Printed in the United States of America

ISBN: 978-0-9820908-0-0

Cover design by S1 GFX 616.617.9904

The author would like to gratefully acknowledge writing consultants Trish Konieczny and E. M. Slootmaker for their invaluable assistance in preparing this book for publication.

Dr. Don VerHulst, MD completed his Doctor of Medicine degree at Wayne State University. Feeling called by the Lord to be a health educator rather than a practicing physician, Dr. Don chose not to become licensed to practice medicine.

dedication

To the One True, Living God

in whom we live and move and have our being!

Acts 17:28; Jeremiah 9:23–24

contents

foreword

Ihave known Dr. Don Ver Hulst for well over twenty years. He was at one time an atheist, then he got saved and set on fire for God. He and Susan have been members of our church for many years, and we have ministered in the States and overseas together.

Dr. Don's approach to biblical health is sound and is very easy to incorporate into your life and family. His book, *Dr. Don's 10 Keys that Cure*, is filled with biblical principles that have been a blessing to Jeanie and me and to our family. I know they will bless you and your family as well.

Duane Vander Klok
Senior Pastor, Resurrection Life Church, Grandville, MI
Founder, Resurrection Life Church International

introduction

God wants you to enroll in His perfect health plan

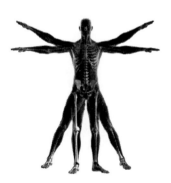

take care of your "earth suit"

Are you familiar with the story about the scientist determined to scale the Mountain of Truth? He acquired all the knowledge humanly possible and struggled mightily through untold hardships to reach the summit, only to find when he got there that a theologian was already sitting on the peak. The scientist had nearly killed himself with his efforts, but the theologian wasn't even out of breath.

I am familiar with that story because I was that scientist. Early on I decided that through knowledge and effort I could give my life meaning and make other people's lives better, so I applied to medical school. I spent years in intensive study and sacrificed myself to a grueling schedule. In 1982 I earned my M.D.

God created us as three-part beings: spirit, soul, and body. All three parts of me were a terrible mess by the time I finished medical school. I was an atheist without any spiritual hope. My mind was filled with medical jargon and tradition. I lived on caffeine, junk food, and adrenaline. I was rail-thin, couldn't gain weight, and I never exercised or got enough rest. I was a living contradiction in terms—a doctor who didn't take care of his health. Despite my sorry physical and spiritual state, I was convinced that I was well on my way to reaching the pinnacle of my life. Then my car battery died one night and the scientist met the theologian.

"What do you believe in?"

It was 4:00 a.m. and freezing cold as I sat in the parking lot of the Detroit Metropolitan Airport trying to start my car. It was hopeless, but before long a gentleman with a truck approached and offered to jumpstart it. He got out his jumper cables and offered to let me sit in his warm vehicle while he charged the dead battery. Once the cables were hooked up he climbed in, too. Out of the blue he asked me a question I wasn't expecting: "What do you believe in?"

An odd question for the middle of the night in a frozen parking lot, but I thought, *Well, this guy's jumping my car battery, so if he wants to talk about the cost of tea in China, all right then, let's talk!* I answered him, "I've heard about God and Jesus, but I don't believe all that. I'm an atheist."

That statement usually either riled people up or scared them into silence, but this late-night theologian was a beautiful witness. I believe he acted just like Jesus would have. First he listened to all I had to say. Then, he asked me a simple question, "Have you ever sinned?"

It took me only a second to reply, "Oh yeah! I'm the grand champion sinner!" (Isn't it interesting that I was an atheist and I still knew I'd sinned? God had been working in my heart.)

"Would you like to be forgiven for your sins?" he asked.

"You mean every wrong thing I've ever done would just be gone?" I asked.

"That's right. Would you like that?"

That's not even remotely possible, I thought. *We're playing a hypothetical game here, but at least my car battery's charging...* So I answered him, "You'd have to be a fool not to want that! Who wouldn't want that?"

> *It was such a revelation that the God of the universe knew all about me—all about each of us—and that He had a specific plan for me.*

"Ask Jesus to come into your heart and be Lord of your life," he suggested.

As an atheist, I had no idea how to pray, but suddenly I knew this guy was sitting on the truth I'd been struggling to reach. I responded with just one word, "Yes." I meant it with my whole heart.

Immediately, the God whom I hadn't even believed in a split-second before, spoke to me as clearly as I've ever heard anyone in my life. "Every word of the

Bible is true," He said. Then He added, "Even the hairs of your head are all numbered."

God was reminding me of a Bible verse I'd heard as a little boy, "The very hairs of your head are all numbered" (Matthew 10:30). It was such a revelation that the God of the universe knew all about me—all about each of us—and that He had a specific plan for me.

For the next three years, all I wanted to do was study God's Word.

the scientific bible

The more I studied the Bible, the more particular Scriptures would jump out at me, especially verses containing divine principles about the physical body, health, and healing. In all my years of medical studies, the Bible was certainly the last book I thought of as a text on physiology. I soon found out, though, that God's Word is absolutely the most current, most accurate text on every subject— including physiology and all the sciences.

> *The more scientists and medical experts discover about our "earth suits," these bodies we have while we're on this planet, the more amazed they are at how the Bible's physiological statements keep proving true.*

The more scientists and medical experts discover about our "earth suits," these bodies we have while we're on this planet, the more amazed they are at how the Bible's physiological statements keep proving true. Every divine principle Scripture has stated about physical health and healing is steadfastly accurate.

In the academic arena I come from, the exact opposite is the case. Medical advice changes all the time—year to year and even month to month. The simplest questions, such as whether a person should take an aspirin daily for heart health, are hotly debated.

I was so glad to find that God's Word provides a rock-solid foundation that doesn't shift constantly. It covers every area of life. As a physician, I was particularly interested to discover that it provides a pattern for good health. I am continually amazed at the simplicity and practicality of God's health plan for us. The Scriptures contain a blueprint we can easily follow to build health and healing in our physical bodies.

My desire is still to have my life count for something—in God's Kingdom—and to benefit other people with what I've learned. That's why I travel, teach, and write about God's perfect health plan for us. I want everyone to enjoy the blessing of good health! Good health is vitally important as we live the abundant life God promises. It enables us to accomplish His purpose. I'm here to tell you that you can enjoy the good health Scripture talks about. God's simple but wonderful health plan will work for you.

That word *health* in the Hebrew means "medicine." God's Word is medicine to your body, soul, and spirit. His divine principles will help you live—really live—and be bursting with health! Trust me as a physician, the medicine we are about to take from His Word is the very best that's available to promote your physical health. And, it's not at all hard to take!

good health in God's word

When I refer to the abundant life in regard to your health, I mean more than just the absence of disease. Good health means being full of vibrant energy and an enthusiasm for living. Christians who take care of their earth suits wake up in the morning full of life not only spiritually, but also physically. They have a spring in their step, and they overflow with the energy needed to go out and do God's will.

The more I studied Scripture from a physician's perspective, the more I saw a blueprint emerge that we can follow to build up and enjoy good health. God's blueprint for our health is wonderful in its simplicity, yet profound in its design. Simple yet profound may sound a bit cliché, but it sums up the perfect health plan God provides us in His Word.

Many people give up on experiencing good health because it seems there are too many rules to follow, too many activities to avoid, and too much involved in setting up a biblical nutrition plan. Feeling guilty about their physical condition, yet completely over-whelmed, many people decide that pursuing good health is just too complicated.

> *Many people give up on experiencing good health because it seems there are too many rules to follow, too many activities to avoid, and too much involved in setting up a biblical nutrition plan.*

My purpose is to reach people with the message that God's simple yet profound health plan *will work* for them. Rather than wrestling with complicated programs or agonizing over all the things they shouldn't do or shouldn't eat, people can get healthy and stay healthy by what I like to call *"doing the do's."* Rather than focusing on the negatives, people who do the do's—the simple things the Bible promotes for good health—reap a huge harvest of physical benefits.

why do the do's?

Your body is *by far* your most valuable worldly possession. You can have five homes, a cottage, a castle, and a yacht, but if you don't have your body, you can't live in any of them! And if you don't have a body, you can't serve the Lord here on earth either. That's why taking care of your body is such an important part of serving Him.

The apostle Paul urged in Romans 12:1, "I beseech you therefore, brethren, by the mercies of God, that you present your bodies a living sacrifice, holy, acceptable to God, which is your reasonable service."

Romans 12:1, "I beseech you therefore, brethren, by the mercies of God, that you present your bodies a living sacrifice, holy, acceptable to God, which is your reasonable service."

Paul also told us in 1 Corinthians 6:13 that our bodies are for the Lord and the Lord is for our bodies. One translation of that verse says "the Lord cares about our bodies" (NLT). I'm glad He cares! It's good to have Him on our side when it comes to health. Many times the Gospels relate that Jesus healed *all* the sick that were brought to Him, and whenever a sick person professed the belief that Jesus could heal *if* He were willing, Jesus always replied, "I am!" It's good to know that "Jesus Christ is the same yesterday, today, and forever" (Hebrews 13:8) and that He still wants us healed, whole, and feeling great.

Why else should we do the do's? They keep us out of trouble! "Blessed is the man whom You instruct, O LORD, and teach out of Your law, that You may give him rest from the days of adversity" (Psalm 94:12–13). When we apply the principles Scripture contains about our health, we are kept from the adversity of serious illness and pain.

"Blessed is the man whom You instruct, O LORD, and teach out of Your law, that You may give him rest from the days of adversity" (Psalm 94:12–13).

"The way of transgressors is hard," warns Proverbs 13:15 (KJV)—those who transgress scriptural health principles and neglect their earth suits will be the first to tell you so. Anyone with a debilitating illness brought on by self-neglect or anyone undergoing a serious operation to correct a problem they could have prevented with healthier living habits will assure you that the trouble they're in just wasn't worth it. They'd do it differently if they could only do it over again!

the health equation

My very first day in medical school, I sat in a classroom of eager young medical students facing our first instructor in our first lecture. "Before I was a physician, I was an engineer," he began, "and when I was an engineer and a machine broke down, I had to go out and fix it. Then we tried the machine, and if it worked I got the credit."

We weren't sure what that statement had to do with medicine. Thankfully, he went on to explain: "Then I became a physician, and as a physician, when the "machine" of the human body breaks down, I watch the machine fix itself—and I still get the credit!"

It's so true. I've seen it over and over again. We are indeed marvelously, wonderfully made (see Psalm 139:14). Our bodies do fix themselves. They are naturally designed to function efficiently, fight off disease, and repair themselves when necessary.

We are already built to enjoy great health—but we, too, have a part to play. Thomas Edison, another brilliant man, recognized this when he said, "The doctor of the future won't prescribe medications for his patients, but he'll educate his patients in the care of the human frame and in the cause and prevention of disease."

If we do our part to care for our human frames the biblical way, we give our bodies what they need to function well and to fight off and prevent disease. That's precisely what I teach people to do, and the first thing I teach is what I call the health equation:

Detoxification + Balancing the Immune System = Great Health

If we will attend to those two areas, detoxification and balancing the immune system, we will become far healthier and stay that way. Detoxification, detox for short, simply means keeping junk out of our bodies and cleansing it of any junk already inside. It's important to "cleanse ourselves from everything that contaminates and defiles body and spirit" (2 Corinthians 7:1, AMPLIFIED). That way, we're best equipped to serve God and carry out His plans for us. In the chapters that follow, we'll suggest positive steps to take to detox and "dejunk" by focusing on great, God-made foods.

Balancing the immune system is also crucial because the immune system both fights off and prevents disease. An immune system strengthened and built up by good health habits can handle any kind of attack that comes at your body, whether it's from an outside source like a virus or an inside source like cancer cells.

waging war on disease

The tools I recommend are 10 keys the Lord showed me about health as I began to study Scripture from a physician's perspective. I call them "Dr. Don's 10 Keys that Cure."

ten keys that cure

The 10 Keys that Cure gleaned from the pages of God's Word can benefit everyone, well or ill.

If you already enjoy good health, they will safeguard it and ensure that you continue enjoying it. If you are sick, they will help you detoxify your body and stabilize your immune system so you can begin to balance the health equation in your favor.

In the next chapters, we'll identify these 10 important keys and examine each one more closely. We'll discover how easy they are to learn and apply, and we'll discuss the specific "do's" you can do to put them into practice. These 10 Keys that Cure are modeled throughout both the Old Testament and New, and we'll observe how Jesus Himself followed them in His daily routines. My hope and prayer for you is that as you follow them, you, too, will reap the blessing of the great health you were meant to enjoy according to the Word of God.

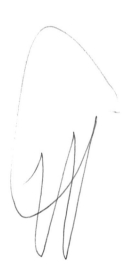

ten keys that cure

Key 1

Learn to Relax Like the Lord

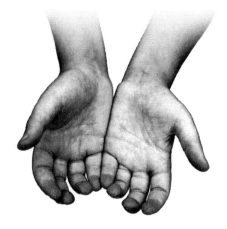

"Learn to relax" is the first and one of the most important of my 10 Keys that Cure. Stress is arguably the number one enemy of the immune system. By stress, I don't mean money troubles, issues with your boss or arguments with your spouse. Those are stressors. Stress is your body's reaction to these stressors.

God instilled in you both a sympathetic nervous system and a parasympathetic nervous system. The latter is the "resting system" that slows your heart rate and helps you relax. The former, the sympathetic nervous system, governs your fight-or-flight reactions to stressors. It can stress your body by increasing your heart rate, blood

It's good to have a bodily system set up to help you survive, and we all need that in certain situations. However, you were never designed to run on continual red alert.

pressure, respiration, nutritional needs, and hormonal activity, all in response to some stimuli or stressor. The body goes on red alert when your fight-or-flight system kicks in. It's good to have a bodily system set up to help you survive, and we all need that in certain situations. However, you were never designed to run on continual red alert.

A couple things happen during a sympathetic nervous system reaction that are not good for your body over the long term. Your body thinks it needs to focus on *survival*, so it temporarily neglects other important functions—at least the reaction is *meant* to be temporary. Your body doesn't think it has time to digest your food properly, so you don't get all the nutrition you need. Your body neglects your immune system because it isn't focusing on fighting cancer, infections, and traumas, it's focusing on your survival. Your body releases fight-or-flight hormones like adrenaline to aid you in your struggle for survival.

No one was designed to continually undergo those kinds of

> *Have you ever heard the saying "you can't live on adrenaline?" It's true; a continual adrenaline rush will put your health into a downhill slide.*

bodily reactions. Have you ever heard the saying "you can't live on adrenaline?" It's true; a continual adrenaline rush will put your health into a downhill slide. Yet myriads of people run around in a highly stressed state day after day.

Our modern lifestyles set us up to live that way, and before long we think it's normal—until it negatively affects our health.

"I have to guard against falling into that trap," Susan says. For a long time she worked outside the home as a popular DJ at a local Christian radio station, and we had little ones too (and still do). "I woke up on the run," she says. "I ran out the door; made sure the kids were cared for; ran to work to record a program, then ran to the studio in the mall. I quick ran to the carwash after work and the grocery store after that, then I ran and got the kids. At home they'd start asking, 'What are we going to do? Let's do this . . . let's do that,' and we'd be off and running again. It's easy to get overstressed and forget about the Sabbath rest—or resting in God at all. Even now, my husband will just look at me as I race around, then he'll ask if I've prayed about whatever's on my mind and on my plate. It stops me cold. We forget to come to God with our burdens and our busyness because we're trying to do it all, and it's making many of us sick!"

One reason I married Susan was because of her high-energy enthusiasm for life. Back in college, part of her energy came from caffeine-laden Cokes and sugar-laden Hostess Sno Balls (those round, pink cakes that come two in a pack), so she was no better than me about balanced nutrition. Now, though, we both attempt to eat God-made foods to produce the energy we need, and we'll talk more about that. We also attempt to *relax*, and for some of us that's harder than for others.

Four-Six It!

How do you relax? I advise people to four-six it. Philippians 4:6 outlines the biblical approach to stress relief: "Be anxious for nothing, but in everything by prayer and supplication, with thanksgiving, let your requests be made known to God." I

Be anxious for nothing, but in everything by prayer and supplication, with thanksgiving, let your requests be made known to God.

love how God not only tells us what not to do, He also tells us what to do! He says let *your* requests be made known—you get to choose your requests, so go ahead and tell Him what you need.

That's a novel idea for many. You'd be surprised how many people look at me like a calf at a new gate when I ask them, "Have you made your requests known to God?" It's a wonderful stress buster. Try it! It will settle you down, as the MESSAGE version of Philippians 4:6–7 promises:

> Don't fret or worry. Instead of worrying, pray. Let petitions and praises shape your worries into prayers, letting God know your concerns. Before you know it, a sense of God's wholeness, everything coming together for good, will come and settle you down. It's wonderful what happens when Christ displaces worry at the center of your life.

Continual anxiety or worry is so hard on your physiological system—not to mention the rest of you! The crazy thing about worry is that a lot of the scenarios we worry about never even come to pass. John Wayne, the no-nonsense tough guy who always seemed so cool and collected in the roles he played, was reported to say, "I've been through a lot of terrible things in my life, some of which actually happened."

That's true for many of us. We concentrate on a thousand what-ifs, leaving ourselves much less time and energy to deal with the realities of life. By worrying, we put ourselves through things mentally and emotionally that might never even happen. And physiologically, our bodies don't know if the stressors we're dwelling on are happening or not. The body's negative reaction to stress is the same either way. That's why worrying can make us sick.

Let's take a minute to do a little stress-relief by four-sixing it right now. It's the most immune system-stimulating, health-giving activity I know of, so give this a try: Prop this book open somehow and put your hands out in front of you, palms up. Visualize all your worries, all the "stuff" in your life, all the "junk in your trunk" as my pastor says, all you're praying about, and all you forgot to pray about in a pile in your hands. Toss *everything* in there (some of us will have a bigger pile than others). On the count of three, lift both hands toward heaven, "casting all your care upon Him, for He cares for you" (1 Peter 5:7). One, two, three . . . offer your cares to God and don't put your hands down until you're sure they're empty! Believe in His perfect will in all your circumstances, and don't bring that pile of cares back to earth again. Leave them at His feet where they belong.

I promise you, your immune system is working better right now than it was a minute ago. You probably feel better too. You can four-six it anytime, as often as you want! People may think you've lost your mind when they see you throwing your hands up to heaven, but that's okay—you have the mind of Christ. Whenever you four-six it, you're following the biblical approach to stress-relief and strengthening your immune system.

Joy Equals Strength

Another relaxation technique is so simple people miss it, yet it's so foundational. Be joyful. That's it. Rejoice in life. "Don't be dejected and sad, for the joy of the Lord is your strength!"

(Nehemiah 8:10, NLT). The Bible equates joy with strength, so if you want to be strong in your immune system, and every other area, let the Lord fill you with His joy.

Refuse to allow joy killers into your life. Your own words are vital in this—"a man has joy by the answer of his mouth" (Proverbs 15:23). Or you have the opposite—your words can bring you sorrow. Align your words with God's Word and speak *positively*. Some people think they're praying when they're really complaining, but realize that God already knows every problem you face. He already has an answer and a plan, so instead of telling God about your problems, tell your problems about God.

Jesus told us to speak *to* the mountains in our lives, not talk about them. Tell your mountain to be removed in Jesus' name (see Matthew 17:20). If you knew what wonders God has waiting for you on the other side, you'd move your mountain in a hurry. Besides, mountains know other mountains, so if you don't tell your mountain to be removed, pretty soon you have a mountain range, right? One you may have built with your own complaints or negative words. It's much better to use the positive approach and be joyful.

Remember there is joy in laughter, so laugh a lot. "A merry heart does good, like medicine" (Proverbs 17:22). Doctors always like that verse since it implies that medicine does good—

"A merry heart does good, like medicine" (Proverbs 17:22).

and sometimes medicine can do good, so long as it's taken with your Gos-pills (the gospel message of the good news). Look at the AMPLIFIED translation: "A happy heart is good medicine and a cheerful mind works healing, but a broken spirit dries up the bones." Don't walk around crushed and broken when there's healing in Jesus Christ for your every wound. Cheer up at that thought, for a cheerful mind works healing! "Rejoice in the Lord always: and again I say, Rejoice" (Philippians 4:4, KJV).

Cast your cares up to heaven and cultivate a joyful heart. In other words, chill out and cheer up! Learning to relax is the first and foremost key to good health. God holds you in the palm of His hand, and He is always on your side. It's the devil who comes to steal, kill, and destroy. Jesus came so that you could enjoy abundant life to the fullest! (See John 10:10.)

Simple Yet Profound: Laugh unto the Lord

In our healing class at church, we sometimes do "laughter therapy" because laughter breaks down a major stress hormone. Stress hormones bathe our brains in acid, and most of us experience enough issues without having acidic brains that deteriorate quickly and give place to all kinds of diseases. So we practice laughing our way into joy. Sometimes we start with a laugh of faith, but that's all right, it works. Try it. Do five seconds of laughter therapy now, and it will probably turn into at least thirty seconds or more. Once you start, joy just bubbles up inside, and you'll feel better afterward.

Around our busy household, it's gotten so I recognize my wife's laugh of faith now. I'll hear Susan's "ha-ha-ha" coming from some other part in the house, and it'll make me start to laugh because I know she's trying to make the best of something that's probably not very funny. I get into agreement with her, and so do the kids! One time, grape juice went flying all over the kitchen table, the curtains, and the floor, and I heard Susan's halfhearted "ha-ha-ha" coming from that direction. The kids probably were thinking *We're in for it now!* After a shocked second, I heard them all join in, "ha-ha-ha, ha-ha-ha!" No doubt they thought keeping Mom laughing was a better alternative than giving her a quiet minute to survey the disaster area.

Laughter breaks your focus from your problems and literally strengthens every system, cell, and organ in your body. My kids know it covers a multitude of sins--even splattering grape juice all over the kitchen. It's amazing that the average adult laughs only 15 times a day, while the average child laughs between 200 and 400 times. My kids laugh all the time. They're full of joy! That keeps their stress hormones from acidifying their brains. A joyful spirit is healthy and healing. Even outside the church, people are laughing themselves into wellness now that researchers have discovered a link between humor and healing.

Key 2

Get to Bed on Time

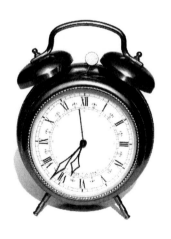

In my classes and seminars, when I bring up the second key to good health, *get to bed on time*, people often start laughing. I think they're going back to key number one and trying to use laughter therapy to overcome the stress they feel about not getting enough sleep.

Rest time is restoration time, and these days most of us have no idea what it's like to wake up feeling restored after a proper night's rest. I cannot overemphasize the simple yet profound benefits of a good night's sleep.

It's hard to get across how vitally important getting to bed on time is, but maybe this statistic will help: Actuarial figures from insurance companies show that people who go longer than seven days on five hours or fewer of sleep a night increase their risk of death from all causes by 700 percent! That's an astronomical increase.

> *People who go longer than seven days on five hours or fewer of sleep a night increase their risk of death from all causes by 700 percent!*

It has also been shown that people who sleep fewer than six hours a night don't live as long as people who sleep seven or more hours. As I said at the start, neglecting your earth suit may not keep you out of heaven, but it will send you there sooner! Not getting sufficient rest can literally kill you.

People who drive while fatigued often don't live long at all! "Driving under the influence" of sleep deprivation can be as dangerous as driving under the influence of alcohol—in fact, after 24 hours of sleeplessness, you are just as impaired behind the wheel of a car as if you were legally drunk! And it doesn't even take 24 hours for sleep deprivation to begin affecting your driving ability. That can start to happen after 17 sleepless hours.

Our bodies require between six and eight hours of good rest every night, and consistency and timing make a world of difference in how you feel and how you function when you wake up in the morning. Studies show that the hours from 10 p.m. until 2 a.m. are the most healing, restorative hours to rest—don't miss those hours of sleep. From 10 p.m. until midnight your sleep is *four times* more restorative than the hours you sleep after midnight, so try especially hard not to miss those hours.

It's worth noting that your stomach needs good rest every night too. If you get plenty of sleep but still wake up tired, maybe you aren't letting your stomach rest when you rest. Have you ever noticed that eating a big meal right before bedtime can disturb your rest or even keep you awake at night? Don't load up your stomach before bed so that it has to keep working hard all night to digest your late-night snacks. Instead, follow the maxim "Eat like a king at breakfast, a prince at lunch, and a pauper at dinner." It will do your stomach and your sleep habits a world of good.

In 1735, Ben Franklin cited another maxim in his almanac: "Early to bed and early to rise, makes a man healthy, wealthy, and wise." That still makes good sense to me. God made it easy for us to figure out when to sleep and when to rise. He gave the sun's bright light to the daytime and the lesser lights of the moon and stars to the night. When God's bright light goes down for

Psalm 127:2 says God "gives His beloved sleep."

the night, you go down. When it rises, you rise.

Ben Franklin was right—it's healthy and wise to sleep when God meant us to sleep. Psalm 127:2 says God "gives His beloved sleep." The AMPLIFIED version says He gives blessings to His beloved in their sleep. Beloved child of God, He can't give you sleep and bless you in it if you won't go to bed!

God Took Time for R & R

So far we have covered the first two Keys that Cure, *learn to relax* and *get to bed on time*. You follow in God's footsteps if you are doing those two things. God Himself takes time for R & R. Genesis, the first book of the Bible, tells us so. God finished His creative works on earth in six days, then He checked them over, saw that they were good, and "He rested on the seventh day from all His work which He had done. And God blessed (spoke good of)

> *He rested on the seventh day from all His work which He had done.*

the seventh day, set it apart as His own, and hallowed it, because on it God rested from all His work" (Genesis 2:2–3, AMPLIFIED).

Some people feel guilty if they take time for R & R, whether that means getting enough sleep at night or allowing for a day of rest on the weekends. Stress, financial worries, or the hectic pace of modern life so overwhelms them that they cannot slow down enough to let their bodies (not to mention their minds and spirits) be restored. God "spoke good of" that seventh day of rest, though, and later, in the Ten Commandments, He instructed Moses and the Israelites to keep holy the Sabbath as well by resting from all their work.

God felt so strongly about R & R that He declared the Sabbath holy and decreed, "Whoever does any work on the Sabbath day, he shall surely be put to death" (Exodus 31:15). If that law were in effect today, we'd all be dead. However, it illustrates how crucial R & R is. If God Himself took time for it and made it law for His chosen people, the Israelites, don't you think we ought to make it a priority as well? We'll actually be more productive in body, mind, and spirit if we are properly rested.

Jesus knew the importance of R & R. He had a whole world

to save, yet look what He did: "Now in the morning, having risen a long while before daylight, He went out and departed to a solitary place; and there He prayed" (Mark 1:35). This one verse contains a whole health seminar, so let's take a closer look at it. You've probably heard the saying "What would

> *You've probably heard the saying "What would Jesus do?" Here's a saying I like better: "Do what Jesus did."*

Jesus do?" Here's a saying I like better: "Do what Jesus did." Do the do's, as Jesus did in this one verse, and you'll go a long way toward experiencing great biblical health.

First, this verse indicates to me that Jesus got to bed on time. How do I know? You don't get up early unless you get to bed on time, and Jesus consistently got up early. He also consistently went to a solitary place, a peaceful place where he could be alone with God, and prayed. Making time for yourself is vital in learning to relax. You need some time alone and some time with just you and God. That's the best kind of R & R!

Notice a couple other things about Jesus' morning routine. The passage in Mark says He rose up and went out—that is, He exercised His physical body. He could have talked to His heavenly Father while lying on His sleeping mat (or wherever He slept; Scriptures tell us sometimes He had nowhere to lay His head). Instead, He got out of bed and took a walk. He walked until He found a peaceful place outside, breathed in the fresh air, and prayed until the sun came up. I think He must have watched many glorious sunrises while He prayed. The disciples came and found Him, so it must have gotten light as he prayed.

Did you notice how Jesus modeled the next three Keys that Cure? He got some exercise, breathed fresh air, and enjoyed the sunshine, the three things we're going to look at in the next chapter. Notice that Jesus was in the habit of ministering to His

entire being. He restored His physical body as He slept, He
exercised, and He got fresh air and sunshine. He restored His
mind (learned to relax) by finding a peaceful place of solitude,
far from the usual press of the crowds. He restored His spirit by
communicating one-on-one with God.

Remember, we are three-part beings: body, soul (mind, will,
and emotions), and spirit. Like Jesus, we need restoration in all
those areas. Jesus painted us a beautiful picture in Mark 1:35
of how to get healthy and stay healthy. Notice one last thing.
His healthy habits enabled Him to accomplish the work God
set before Him. When the disciples found Him that morning
and informed Him that everyone was looking for Him, Jesus
was refreshed and ready to minister again. The disciples were
probably ready to walk back with Him and eat breakfast, but
Jesus had much bigger plans. "Let's go to the rest of the villages
so I can preach there also. This is why I've come," He told them.
Then look what He did: "He went to their meeting places all
through Galilee, preaching and throwing out the demons" (Mark
1:38–39, MESSAGE).

Sounds like Jesus had more than enough energy to fulfill
God's call. Let's take a look at those next three keys and see how
we can be more like Him.

Simple Yet Profound: Why Can't You Sleep?

Menopause, sleep apnea and restless legs.

As you age, several factors can cause your sleep quantity and
quality to suffer. For women, menopausal hot flashes and night
sweats can interrupt sleep. However, recent studies indicate that
menopausal women are also likely to suffer from two other age-
related sleep problems: sleep apnea and restless leg syndrome
(RLS). Having a healthy body weight can help with sleep apnea.
Your doctor may also recommend therapeutic devices to help

you keep your airway open. RLS may respond to improved nutrition, vitamin and iron supplementation, regular exercise, and removing caffeine and alcohol from your daily routine.

Mind over matters.

Many of us also suffer from RMS--restless mind syndrome! You are so tired, that bed feels so good, but your brain just won't shut up. One way to quiet the mind is through quiet prayer and reflection on God's word before you retire. As an herbal adjunct, try a nice hot cup of green tea with lemon balm. Green tea has an amino acid, L-Theanine, that helps your brain produce soothing alpha waves.

Mellow out with melatonin.

Another factor, imbalanced melatonin production can wreak havoc on your sleep cycle. Melatonin is a hormone that enables deep, healthy sleep. Older folks tend to produce less melatonin than they need at night and more during the day when it causes drowsiness. Sleeping in total darkness can help restore a balanced melatonin production schedule. Melatonin is also available in supplemental form.

The half-night sleep.

Do you find it easy to fall asleep only to awake a few hours later to an agonizing sleepless night? This type of sleep pattern deprives you of the several complete sleep cycles you need to maintain good health. Even a nap during the day can't make up for losing sleep at night. The ancient herb valerian may help you get to sleep and stay asleep. Valerian increases the levels of the amino acid GABA in your system. GABA induces sleep while helping to regulate relaxation and anxiety.

Medications and illnesses.

If you are taking a prescription for blood pressure or seizures or are using antidepressants, diuretics or stimulants (diet pills or amphetamines), you may have trouble getting a good night's sleep. Talk to your doctor. Heart disease, respiratory disease, GI problems and endocrine disease are just a few ailments that can also interfere with your sleep cycle.

Key 3

Faith is a Moving Experience: Exercise

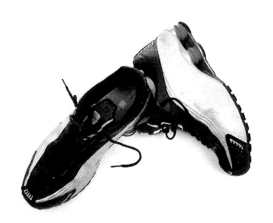

Horses were for the rich or the Roman in Jesus' day. Scripture refers to people occasionally traveling by boat, but when they were on land they usually walked. Other than riding into Jerusalem on a donkey at Passover, Jesus walked almost everywhere. So did his disciples. They all got their exercise—it was an inescapable part of their daily routine.

Not so for us today. Many of us escape exercise as frequently as we can. We drive to work, sit at our desks all day, then drive home and sit in front of the TV. That's a lot of sitting but not much exercise--unless we count pushing pencils or lifting food to our mouths as exercise. Yet "do your exercise" is my third vital key to good health.

You knew that infamous "E" word, *exercise*, would show up somewhere, didn't you? Jesus exercised every day, and we want to be like Him, right? Only we don't *have to* exercise to get from one place to another, we *get to* exercise for our health.

> *Jesus exercised every day, and we want to be like Him, right?*

Having to do something seems negative; *getting to* do something seems positive. I like to concentrate on the positive, so I always say *get to* instead of *have to*. My kids always see that one coming. I set them up all the time by saying, "You don't *have to* do this, you know . . ."

They don't even let me finish my sentence anymore. "We know, we know, Dad," they answer. "We *get to* do it . . ."

You and I *get to* exercise, so let's think of it as a privilege. If we are able to exercise, it *is* a privilege, an opportunity to reap the blessing of good health. We tend to think we pay such a high price to exercise—an interruption in our day, one more thing to fit into our busy schedule, a little physical discomfort. But in reality we don't pay the price for good health habits—we pay the price for poor health habits. Just ask anyone who is hospitalized if the price they're paying for not exercising, not eating healthy foods, and not taking care of their body was worth it. Their answer will be a thousand times no!

Let's do what Jesus did—walk. The average person in Jesus' time walked three to ten miles a day. Jesus Himself walked well over twenty thousand miles over the course of His ministry!

You and I don't need to end up where they are. We can make simple little changes in our daily routines to incorporate exercise. Let's do what Jesus did— walk. The average person in Jesus' time walked three to ten miles a day. Jesus Himself walked well over twenty thousand miles over the course of His ministry!

I haven't covered twenty thousand miles yet, but walking is my favorite exercise. A brisk walk of thirty to 45 minutes three to five days a week is almost as beneficial as jogging. Or an easier way to think of it is to do the 4:40. That's 40 minutes of walking four times a week. You'll enjoy it more than you think, and it'll make you feel terrific.

Did you know, by the way, that you can exercise your insides? Laughter is your insides jogging. Studies have shown that 5 minutes of belly laughter burns almost as many calories as moderate walking. I like that. I'd rather laugh for 5 minutes than jog five miles any day!

Keep in mind that you don't need to speed along fast, get your heart wildly racing, and run out of breath to make your walking count. It is good, however, to do more than stroll. Whenever I suggest exercising together, Susan will say, "No thanks, that's all right," because I tend to stroll. When Susan walks, she briskly moves along and gets her arms swinging. "If I'm going to do this, I'm going to make it count," she tells me. Meanwhile, I stroll along and tell her I'm four-sixing it, casting all my cares on Him. Susan and I exercise at different paces, but at least we both exercise!

"Bodily exercise profits a little, but godliness is profitable for all things," says 1 Timothy 4:8. In the Greek that verse literally reads, "Bodily exercise profits for a season, but spiritual exercise is profitable eternally." For what season is bodily exercise profitable? For the season that you're in

> *Bodily exercise profits for a season, but spiritual exercise is profitable eternally.*

your body here on earth! You are God's temple, God's mobile home so to speak, and you only get to travel around down here for as long as your body lasts.

It's Never Too Late

Most of us are non-exercisers. Even though we believe in exercise—90 percent of Americans rate exercise as essential to good health. We just don't do it—only 20 percent of Americans actually exercise. If you are among the majority, the non-exercising crowd (and it *is* a crowd), take heart. No matter how old you are or what shape you're in, it's never too late to get moving to help your body last longer and be stronger.

My mom is in her early seventies, and she's in good shape! "If I don't move it, I'll lose it," she says. She lives next door, which makes me like Raymond in *Everybody Loves Raymond*. Sometimes Raymond and I get the short end of the stick, but mostly it's great having Mom next door.

Since Mom is retired and Dad is in Heaven, Mom loves to have the grandkids visit and keep her company, so some mornings our kids walk over to Grandma's. One morning my son walked over and Grandma was exercising while tuned in to fitness expert Denise Austin on TV. Grandma knew Donnie would want to watch a cartoon, so she said he could have the TV as soon as she finished. Donnie sat there half awake, watching Grandma and

Denise Austin. He looked at Grandma exercising, looked at the TV, looked at Grandma again, and said, "You know, Grandma, you're never going to look like her." Mom got a big laugh out of that one!

> *My mother is a beautiful seventy-something! She's sharp, too. Exercisers are three to five times less likely to suffer from Alzheimer's disease.*

Exercise may not restore your youth and beauty, but it will go a long way toward making you feel young and beautiful again. My mother is a beautiful seventy-something! She's sharp, too. Exercisers are three to five times less likely to suffer from Alzheimer's disease.

If you're a non-exerciser, I want to recommend a great move to get you started. The best thing about this move is that you can do it while watching TV (not that I recommend you exercise in front of the TV all the time, but you have to start somewhere). During every commercial, do chair lifts. Have you ever seen weight lifters do squats in a gym? Same principle. Stand up as soon as a commercial starts, then squat down until your back end nearly touches your chair again—but not quite. Then jump up, springing as high as you can with your hands in the air.

Chair lifts work every major muscle group and are aerobic as well. They're a simple move with complex benefits. Do chair lifts as many times as you can during commercials, aiming for a goal of two sets of ten repetitions each during each commercial break. Once you hit that goal, take it to the next level and add a can of soup in each hand for resistance. Imagine the good shape you'd be in if you had done chair lifts for every commercial you'd ever seen. Do them from now on in place of running to the fridge. It won't tale long to notice a big difference in how you look and feel.

The Astonishing Effects of Exercise

Exercise does wonderful things for your body. It releases endorphins, which are "feel-good" neurotransmitters, or brain chemicals, that literally make you feel better. That's why some depression can be treated with consistent exercise. Exercise is also the number one treatment for osteoporosis (thinning of the bones), hypertension (high blood pressure), insomnia (trouble sleeping), and many other ailments.

Studies show that four hours of exercise a week reduces a woman's risk of breast cancer by 60 percent! That alone makes it worth the effort for any woman. In fact, exercise has been shown to reduce the risk of colon cancer, pancreatic cancer, and prostate cancer too. Exercise can also prevent, control, and even *reverse* adult-onset diabetes (because it reduces fat and allows insulin to start working again). Given the high incidence of diabetes these days, that makes exercise worth the effort for anyone. I can't think of one ailment that exercise wouldn't hugely benefit.

Exercise strengthens your heart muscle and increases your circulation or blood flow, too. As God's Word says, "the life of the flesh is in the blood" (Leviticus 17:11). The oxygen-carrying capacity of your body increases as your blood flow increases, and that's good news because all diseases hate oxygen!

Your brain loves oxygen. The more you exercise, the more oxygen reaches your brain, and the better your mental state. Exercise is the one and only thing that will increase your mental alertness and your emotional tranquility/stability with no side effects. Doesn't it sound good to have mental clarity when you need it and also be able to relax and feel peaceful inside? Exercise promotes both!

How about all those people you've heard of who had to have heart bypass surgery? Did you know regular exercise promotes natural bypasses? Your body continually makes collateral

·······································

> *How about all those people you've heard of who had to have heart bypass surgery? Did you know regular exercise promotes natural bypasses?*

arterials, the "alternate routes" for blood flow should the main routes be blocked. Exercise is the only way to consistently increase that collateral circulation; the more you exercise, the more collateral arterials your body makes. Whatever physical problem a person may have, increasing blood flow by way of consistent, moderate exercise can be a vitally important part of the treatment program.

How about migraines? If you've ever been incapacitated by one of those, you know what pain and suffering is. If you are a migraine sufferer, though, I have great news for you. Studies show that increasing your water intake and engaging in consistent, moderate exercise markedly decreases—and often completely eliminates—the incidence of migraines. That spells relief the natural way.

Exercise and the Health Equation

Why are people who consistently exercise healthier? Exercise helps balance the health equation. Remember the health equation mentioned in the introduction? *Detoxification + balancing the immune system = great health.* The immune system moves its contents around your body via the lymphatic system. You generally have three to five times as much lymphatic fluid in your body as you do blood. Your circulatory system has a pump (your heart) that circulates the blood, but your lymphatic system does not have a pump to circulate the lymphatic fluid. It's a passive system that contains one-way valves but no pump, so lymphatic or immune system fluids don't move around inside you very much unless *you* move.

The lymphatic fluid of a sedentary person circulates through his or her body about once a day. In someone who exercises, it circulates through the body three or four times a day. That's a big difference, and that's why people who consistently exercise have stronger immune systems. That lymphatic fluid with its immune-boosting ingredients moves throughout their bodies much more.

Since moving your muscles moves your lymphatic fluids, move *somehow*. If all you can do because of your health issues is walk once around the block, then walk around the block! I had a friend who said all he could do was get up in the morning and walk four times around the block. I thought that was a decent start toward exercising, until he told me that after he finished, he slid the block under his bed and went back to sleep!

> *If all you can do because of your health issues is walk once around the block, then walk around the block!*

Don't start exercising that way, but start. If all you can do when you're sick is move one leg, move that leg! Move whatever you can move to get that immune system fluid circulating.

As an added bonus, exercise also helps the body properly detoxify—you sweat out toxins and tend to drink more water, the ultimate body purifier. Sweating is a fantastic way to detox, but remember that you also sweat out minerals when you work out. As you engage in an exercise program, make sure you replace those minerals you lose with a good supplement. (We'll cover supplements briefly in the final chapter.)

I mentioned already that exercise releases endogenous morphines called endorphins throughout your body. Those act as your body's naturally produced version of painkillers. Have you ever wondered how on earth people who start exercising and stick with it wind up *enjoying* it? Now you know. Regular exercisers experience the pleasant effects of the endorphins released in their systems, and they actually miss exercise and don't feel as well when they skip it. Wouldn't you like to be in that position? You can be if you start exercising and stick with it.

The "W" Word

The infamy of the "E" word, *exercise*, is nothing compared to the infamy of the "W" word, but we might as well cover them both. Are you ready? Don't stop reading when you find out that the "W" word is *weight*. Before you panic, realize that *you are not what you weigh*. By that I mean your health is not dependent on whether you fit within the "normal" weight range for your height on those equally infamous weight charts.

So often we judge ourselves by the scale, but it's not about the numbers. It's about how you feel and how your energy level holds up to whatever God is calling you to do. What you weigh right now means far less to me as a physician than what you're doing for your health on a daily basis. I recommend that you "live it" rather than "di-

> *What you weigh right now means far less to me as a physician than what you're doing for your health on a daily basis.*

et"—instead of buying into every fad diet that comes along and watching your weight bounce up and down like a roller coaster, start doing the do's such as exercising and eating wholesome, God-made foods. Those lifestyle habits will get you to your *ideal* weight eventually and keep you there.

As we travel and teach my 10 Keys that Cure, we meet many people who are very thin yet very unhealthy, the way I was in medical school. We meet people who are at their perfect chart weight yet are unhealthy because they aren't doing the do's. We also meet people who are technically overweight by the charts, yet they are starting to do the right things and they are reaping the benefits.

One of the best things anyone can do to reach ideal weight is exercise. Why does it seem like the "E" word and "W" word always go together? Because exercise builds muscle, and muscle is your best friend when you're trying to reach and maintain your ideal weight. It is crucial to build muscle because a pound of muscle burns forty calories a day—even at rest—just because it exists. A pound of fat burns only a couple calories.

> *Because exercise builds muscle, and muscle is your best friend when you're trying to reach and maintain your ideal weight.*

Muscle is much more efficient than fat. That's the good news. The bad news is that beginning at age twenty, the average person loses one pound of lean muscle mass every year for the rest of his or her life. Take a minute to do the math—in the decade from twenty to thirty years of age, the average person loses ten pounds of lean muscle mass. This means your body burns 400 fewer calories per day at thirty than it did at twenty when you're at rest. Go from thirty to forty years old and that's 800 fewer calories a day. By fifty—and this is really scary because I'm turning fifty as we publish this book—it's up to 1,200 fewer calories. That's 1,200 calories of food I can't eat at fifty without paying a price, though I could have eaten them at twenty!

Keep in mind that such a scary progression doesn't have to happen. It happens for the average non-exercising person, but those who exercise keep their muscle mass from deteriorating. If you didn't want to exercise before, that fact is enough to make you an exercise wannabe. While you're sitting on the couch watching the electronic income reducer, start doing something. During commercials, get going on those chair lifts I talked about and grab a couple cans of soup to do some bicep reps while you're at it. You'll build muscle mass before you know it!

Proverbs 18:9 AMPLIFIED says, "He who does not use his endeavors to heal himself is brother to him who commits suicide." The footnote on the verse says it "squarely addresses

"He who does not use his endeavors to heal himself is brother to him who commits suicide."

the problem of whether one has a moral right to neglect his body by 'letting nature take its unhindered course' in illness." Heaven forbid we should neglect our bodies! God's Word tells us to do our part, so we need to exercise. We have a moral obligation to use our endeavors to heal ourselves. I believe those endeavors should include exercise along with my other Keys to Health.

Statistics show that for every hour you exercise, you add two hours to your life. That's endeavoring to heal yourself. I'll never forget mentioning this statistic at a health club where there was a seventy-five-year-old lady in the front row. She had on a headband and her jogging suit, and she had just finished running five miles. She was on the edge of her seat, soaking up my health presentation, and when she heard this statistic, she piped up, "At that rate, I'll never die!" I still haven't done the math to figure that one out. I do know, though, that for all of us, exercise will certainly help our earth suits last longer.

Simple Yet Profound: Working in a Workout

Hi! Susan here! I know how difficult it can be to work in a workout! After I gave birth to our fourth baby, Vivian, I was discouraged with the out of shape, tired reflection I saw in my mirror every morning. And there were so many clothes in my closet that I couldn't get my baby fat to squeeze into. I knew it was time for me to get back in shape—but the problem was how? I was working part time, taking care of my four babies, supporting Dr. Don in his ministry, plus the laundry, healthy dinners—how could I add yet another activity to my hectic lifestyle?

Well, that's when our faith always comes in handy, am I right? I took it to the Lord in prayer. And He answered my prayer. Right about that time, the company I was working for began offering employees memberships in a nearby gym and fitness club. I took them up on the offer. But even if you don't have the luxury of belonging to a club, you still can work fitness into your life. The Lord wants you to be healthy and He'll help you meet your fitness goals.

Here are some more ways that I work in a workout into my daily schedule.

On the phone

When you're waiting on hold or enjoying a good telephone conversation with a friend, take the opportunity to stretch. Bend at the waist to stretch out the backs of your legs. Twist side-to-side to loosen your back. Tip your head side-to-side to release tension in your neck. Sit down and circle your ankles, clockwise and counterclockwise.

While watching TV

Have hand weights handy so you can do reps while you watch. Curl your hands up towards your body to work biceps. Hold weights in the center and lift with your elbows leading to work upper arms. Hold the weights interlocked behind your head and lift to work off under the arm flab. During commercials, do ten crunches or push-ups.

Morning and night

I always do ten push-ups first thing in the morning and another ten just before I get into bed at night.

Proactive parking

Instead of stressing over finding the closest parking space to the door, park at the very edge of the parking lot and walk a few extra steps.

Of course, working in a more formal workout into your schedule will give you even more benefits. For starters, choose an activity you enjoy. I hate cycling so you won't find me in any of those spinning classes! Choose something that's fun and you'll be more likely to continue.

And, invite a friend to join you. You will not only increase your fun factor, but also provide accountability. If you can't find a friend to join you, join a class and make some new friends!

Key 4

Great Health in the Great Outdoors:
Breathe Fresh Air

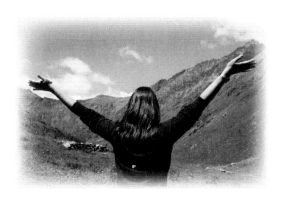

Every cell in your body requires oxygen every second of the day. Oxygen is your cells' number one nutrient. Proper oxygen delivery to every cell of your body is absolutely essential, seeing as all of your body functions depend on breathing.

Some experts believe oxygen deficiency is the single greatest cause of all disease. Deep breathing fights off disease in more than one way. Most importantly, it provides your cells with the oxygen they require to function well and stay healthy. In addition, deep breathing, like exercise, helps move your lymphatic fluid through your body.

> *Some experts believe oxygen deficiency is the single greatest cause of all disease.*

You actually create a vacuum effect inside you when you take a deep breath, which pulls the lymphatic fluid throughout your immune system. Cancer, infection, and diseases of every sort hate oxygen, so fight them off by taking a deep breath of fresh air.

Besides balancing your immune system, deep breathing also enhances detoxification, the other part of the health equation. Deep breathing can increase your body's rate of toxic elimination by as much as fifteen times the normal rate. That's huge!

Deep breathing is a wonderful technique to combat stress. It helps you four-six it (cast all your cares on the Lord). Try this: Breathe in for four seconds, then hold it for four seconds. Breathe out slowly. You just relieved stress. You broke your focus off anything you were going through and took a minute to relax and refresh every cell in your body. You can do that anytime, anywhere.

Breathing happens automatically; you don't even think about breathing as you read these pages. Your respiratory system is another of God's marvelous designs that promote your health. Use it fully, as God intended, and you'll reap huge health benefits. Keep breathing fresh air—it sure beats the alternative!

Simple Yet Profound: Go Smoke Free for God

It goes without saying that my fourth health key, breathing fresh air, leaves no room for smoking. I want to stay focused on the positive things you can do for your health, not a list of "don'ts," but since many people struggle with nicotine, I'll just add a word here I hope will help. If you're a smoker, did you know that if you quit, your potential for improving your health is off the charts? In just two years from the time you stop smoking, 80 percent of the negative changes in your lungs will disappear. That's phenomenal! And further down the road, almost all of smoking's negative effects on your respiratory system will be gone. And you can quit for about 79 cents.

For that price, you can buy a little squeeze bottle of lemon juice at the grocery store. Each and every time you crave a cigarette, put that little bottle in your mouth and give it a good squeeze. It will do a couple things for you. First, the shock will "reset" your system—literally. As your taste buds react to the lemon juice, you'll forget all about your nicotine urge. Second, it will provide some negative conditioning. Most people don't enjoy the taste of lemon juice—an understatement—and you'll start thinking twice before thinking of a cigarette. (If you're one of those rare people who do like lemon juice, then it will provide you with a pleasant diversion from a cigarette instead . . .).

Try the lemon juice method and see what happens. Kicking the nicotine habit will save you money and save your health, not to mention the health of those around you. (We've all heard how horrible the effects of even secondhand smoke can be.) Best of all, it will enable you to breathe fresh air deeply and benefit from it fully, as God intended.

Key 5

Great Health in the Great Outdoors:
Sunshine

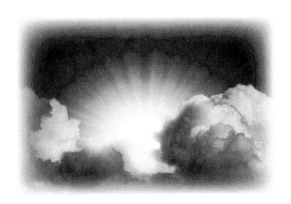

ten keys that *cure*

....

Along with fresh air, sunshine is a major component of good health. Exposure to the sun is my fifth key. I love basking in the sunshine. It makes me feel better.

Granted there need to be wise limits on sun exposure. Nobody wants to suffer horrendous sunburn and its ill effects on health and comfort. However, staying completely out of the sun is much worse for you than exposure in small doses. Avoiding the sun completely or lavishing liberal amounts of sunscreen on yourself every time you step outside is not good for you.

Sunshine is vital to the process of converting cholesterol in your skin into Vitamin D, which promotes strong bones. The bones are where the immune system's cells are formed. No wonder people long to step out into the sunshine when they see it. Go ahead—a little every day is good for you!

How much is good for you? From a practical perspective, to manufacture adequate amounts of vitamin D you need to get out in the sun without sunscreen or long sleeves for 20 minutes at least three times a week. If your skin is dark or if you're older than 65, even more sunshine is required because your production of vitamin D is slower— more like 40 minutes of sunshine three times a week.

Of course, you would be wise to avoid sunburn by working your way up gradually to that amount of exposure. For example, you could choose Mondays, Wednesdays, and Fridays as your "Sundays" and start with 5 minutes of exposure on the first Monday. On Wednesday make it 10 minutes of exposure, and on Friday 15 minutes. In the following weeks continue adding 5 minutes to your exposure time each "Sun-day" until you have worked your way up by 5-minute increments to 40 minutes total sun time.

Another important thing I always do when I go out in the sun, I keep my skin properly hydrated internally and externally. I do this by making sure I drink adequate fluids (8 to 12 glasses of water a day) and by using natural skin moisturizing lotions. I apply these especially after a shower, when it's easiest to trap some of the moisture in the skin. Healthy skin is properly hydrated skin.

Breathe Fresh Air "When the Sun's Out There"

Sunshine is also intimately related to your wake-sleep cycle. The sun's rising and falling sets your circadian rhythm, or your biological clock (not in the reproductive sense, but in the daily functioning of your body). If you never see the light of day, you'll feel like you're in a time warp. Your timing will be off (just ask someone who has been on third shift for a while).

> *Sunshine is also intimately related to your wake-sleep cycle. The sun's rising and falling sets your circadian rhythm*

The way we live today, it's no wonder people frequently suffer from light deprivation disease, or seasonal affective disorder. Never feeling the sun's warm rays or seeing its cheerful light is enough to make anyone feel deprived. Even sitting near a window and letting sunlight hit your eyes is good for you. The sunlight travels through your pupils into your retina and is picked up by your brain, where the impulses go to your pineal gland. That's the master gland that regulates many of your body's other glands, and it is regulated by light and darkness. It secretes melatonin, a hormone linked to strengthening your immune system and setting your circadian rhythm.

Ecclesiastes 11:7 affirms: "Truly the light is sweet, and it is pleasant for the eyes to behold the sun."

God meant for us to enjoy the magnificent sun, as Ecclesiastes 11:7 affirms: "Truly the light is sweet, and it is pleasant for the eyes to behold the sun." It's pleasant, and it's good for you in moderation.

Eat, Drink and Be Healthy!

At this point, we've made it through the first 5 of my 10 Keys that Cure. In the previous chapter we discussed Keys 1 and 2, *Learn to Relax* and *Get to Bed on Time*. In this chapter we covered Keys 3, 4, and 5, *Exercise, Breathe Fresh Air,* and *Sunshine.* Don't you feel better already knowing about these simple things you can do to promote good health?

We've seen in Mark 1:35 that Jesus did these five things, and Ephesians 5:1 tells us we're to "be imitators of God [copy Him and follow His example]" (AMPLIFIED). We need to act like Jesus in regard to our health, doing the do's we've already talked about.

The next chapters will cover my next 5 Keys that Cure, which have to do with what we eat and drink. Our food choices are crucial to our health. We need to eat, drink, and be healthy about it. What food and drink choices should we make when we have an opportunity to choose? What did God intend for us to eat? Why is it true that "you are what you *ate*"? Let's move on and find out.

Simple Yet Profound: Broccoli for Sunscreen?

The more I learn about commercial sunscreens, the more I want to warn my patients about the dangers of overusing them. For one, sunshine is good for you. 20 minutes in the sun on a summer's day provides you with all the Vitamin D you need. If you have dark skin or clothes are covering most of your body, you'll need more time than that.)

Scientists have raised concerns about certain chemicals in sunscreens: diethanolamine, triethanolamine (DEA, TEA), padimate-o, octyl dimethyl PABA, benzophenone, oxybenzone, homosalate, octyl-methoxycinnamate (octinoxate), salicylates and parabens. Some are known carcinogens (cancer causers) and others are hormone benders.

U.S. researchers are working on a new safer sunscreen made from extracts of broccoli sprouts. Their study, published in Proceedings of the National Academy of Sciences, says it works inside your cells by boosting the production of a network of protective enzymes that defend against ultraviolet radiation damage. The effect lasts for several days, even after the extract is no longer present on or in the skin.

Personally, I like wearing my broccoli on the inside. My family loves chomping on it raw to get all the wonderful nutrients that God created. Meanwhile, we get outdoors for fresh air and sunshine! I hope you are, too. It's good for you!

Key 6

Bring Forth Fruit

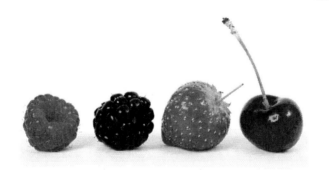

Staying Connected to the Dirt

Eating fruits and vegetables is an excellent route to good health because they keep us connected to the dirt—or more politely, to the dust—from which we are made. Genesis 2:7 says, "And the Lord God formed man of the dust of the ground, and breathed into his nostrils the breath of life; and man became a living being."

> *And the Lord God formed man of the dust of the ground, and breathed into his nostrils the breath of life; and man became a living being.*

The original Hebrew reads "man became another speaking spirit." At the moment God breathed His breath into Adam's nostrils, God's kind of spirit life came alive in humankind.

Now, to stay strong we need to stay connected to where we came from. Spiritually, we need to stay connected to our Source, our Creator. We do that by daily prayer and by staying in His Word. His Word is life and health to us, and those who stay connected to Him stay spiritually strong.

The same is true physically. We need to stay connected to our source, the dirt or dust. Note Genesis 2:7 says the Lord "formed man." To *form* is different than to *create*. God created the heavens and earth—He made something that didn't exist before. When it came to humankind, though, God *formed* man, which means He took something that He had already created, the dust, and molded it into the shape of a man.

"You were made from dust, and to the dust you will return," says Genesis 3:19 (NLT), but in the meantime, we'll be healthiest while we're here if we stay connected to the source of our physical makeup, the ground. We do that by eating what Susan and I call "God-made" foods, the foods God caused to spring up from the

....

earth—the dirt. This divine nutrition principle is so important that God mentions it in the first chapter of the Bible. God caused the earth to bring forth plants and said, "Behold, I have given you every herb bearing seed, which is upon the face of all the earth, and every tree, in the which is the fruit of a tree yielding seed; to you it shall be for meat [or food]" (Genesis 1:29, KJV).

"Herb-bearing seeds" and "fruit-yielding trees" refer to fruits, vegetables, and whole grains. (Key 8 is whole grains, and we'll get to that in the next chapter.) God designed our bodies to function best on these God-made foods, not on man-made foods.

"Behold, I have given you every herb bearing seed, which is upon the face of all the earth, and every tree, in the which is the fruit of a tree yielding seed; to you it shall be for meat [or food]" (Genesis 1:29, KJV).

Plant a seed in rich soil. That seed will reorganize the soil's nutrients and grow into a sprout, then into a mature, food-producing plant. You come along and eat the food that seed produced—you eat reorganized dirt—and you reorganize it into fuel for your body. That process keeps you connected to your physical source. (If an animal comes along and beats you to the produce, then you eat the animal, of course, and still get the benefit of staying connected to where you came from.)

In essence, between the dust we were created from and the produce we eat, we are all reorganized dirt. Don't worry, though, that doesn't make us all dirtbags. .

Follow the Owner's Manual

When an engineer designs something complex such as a car or computer, and you purchase it, you receive an owner's manual that helps you take good care of the product. If you follow the care and maintenance plan laid out in the owner's manual, you'll get long life out of your purchase and it will work well for you. However, if you decide you're smarter than the product's creator and you ignore the instructions in the owner's manual, you'll run into trouble down the road. The product will malfunction and eventually break down completely because you haven't taken proper care of it.

Your car won't run smoothly if you never change the oil. Your computer will crash if you never update the virus protection. Likewise, your body will break down if you don't feed it the foods it needs to maintain good health. Your body is, as we said, your most important earthly possession. Doesn't it make sense, then, to put into practice what you read in your body's "owner's manual"?

> *I consider God's Word the owner's manual for humankind. Written by the Engineer who created us, it gives us detailed care and maintenance instructions...*

I consider God's Word the owner's manual for humankind. Written by the Engineer who created us, it gives us detailed care and maintenance instructions for all three parts of our makeup— body, soul (mind, will, and emotions), and spirit. Following the Bible's instructions about how to care for ourselves, and each other, seems like common sense to me.

For example, God's Word tells us to four-six it and cast all our cares on Him (Philippians 4:6). I know I am stronger spiritually when I four-six it. It also tells us that we are to have the mind of Christ (1 Corinthians 2:16) and that God has given us a sound mind (2 Timothy 1:7). My mind works more clearly and my emotions are more stable when I follow God's principles.

Regarding our physical maintenance, Jesus modeled my first five Keys that Cure in Mark 1:35. Also, God specifically told us what to eat in Genesis 1:29. Many other Scriptures refer to food, but that verse is our Designer's first mention of what we are to eat. You've perhaps already heard of the Genesis diet. Genesis 1:29 is the foundation on which that nutritional plan is built. It's a strong foundation for physical health!

> *Susan and I make sure that about 50 percent of our family's food intake comes from the fruits and vegetables God ordained for us to eat.*

Susan and I make sure that about 50 percent of our family's food intake comes from the fruits and vegetables God ordained for us to eat. You may be thinking, *That's a lot of tomatoes and cucumbers, and I'm not fond of either one!* Many people feel that way. We've also met a lot of people who either love fruits and hate vegetables or hate fruits and love vegetables. In any case, it helps to remember God loves variety. He created a seemingly endless variety of plants and animals for us to discover and explore. Fruits and vegetables come in every shape, size, color, and taste. When was the last time you explored the taste of a new fruit or vegetable or tried a new way of preparing one you thought you didn't like?

Apples, Oranges, Bananas . . .

One nutritious food that promotes all-around great health is fruits. I may be in a classroom full of school children, or in my adult health and healing classes at church, or giving a seminar as a guest speaker, but wherever I am, I always sing to my students about fruit. Sometimes they think I'm fruity, especially when I sing this verse of the "10 Keys" song:

> *Apples, oranges, bananas,*
> *Bright colors you can see,*
> *These are the keys to nutrition,*
> *Your body will agree.*

Fruits are attractive because they are often brightly colored. The depth of color to a fruit (or vegetable) roughly indicates how nutrient rich it is, so the brighter, the better! Fruits also usually taste sweet. They are the kinds of sweets you can really enjoy! Jesus enjoyed them. Look at Mark 11:12: "Now the next day, when they had come out from Bethany, He [Jesus]was hungry. And seeing from afar a fig tree having leaves, He went to see if perhaps He would find something on it."

"Now the next day, when they had come out from Bethany, He [Jesus]was hungry. And seeing from afar a fig tree having leaves, He went to see if perhaps He would find something on it."

When Jesus was hungry, He looked for fruit like figs. Have you tasted them? (Not Fig Newton cookies—I mean the real thing!) Figs are really a seed pod. Research has shown that their seeds contain powerful minerals that fight cancer and all manner of disease. Their nutrients also help keep your circulatory system clean and strengthen your immune system.

Bananas also are excellent too because they most closely parallel the mineral content of the human body. When you eat a banana, you're eating what you're mostly made of. Just about everything you need mineral-wise is conveniently packaged inside that banana peel, so make it a habit to peel back a banana every day. (Make sure to properly dispose of the wrapper, though, or your health might slip away.)

To get our kids excited about eating fruit, we get excited. We say, "Guess what?!? We have—you won't believe this—we have *blueberries* and *watermelon*!" The kids get all excited and start shouting because they think watermelon and blueberries mean a party. Habits are as much caught as taught, so if you get excited about eating fruit, so will your kids. Kids basically do as you do, not as you say, so you need to set the example and eat your fruits with some enthusiasm. We've been having watermelon/blueberry parties since our kids were small. There's nothing like bringing a huge, green watermelon home from the store on a hot summer day! Not to mention watermelon is a natural diuretic. It really helps you get in your 8 to 12 glasses of water in a day.

We also enjoy eating cherries—Michigan, where we live, is famous for its production of sweet black cherries. Cherry Festival time is a real celebration. Did you know cherries are especially effective in combating arthritis and gout? Cranberries are another great fruit. They're well-known for their ability to combat kidney and bladder infections because of their antimicrobial activity and high vitamin C content.

Susan and the children love to put these and other fruits in cereal or in oatmeal with a touch of real maple syrup and a dash of cinnamon. Susan also tops whole grain pancakes and waffles with fruit and real maple syrup—breakfast doesn't get any more healthy or delicious than that!

Another fruit my wife loves is grapefruit. Susan gets more excited about finding just the right color pink grapefruit than most people get about eating a perfectly cooked steak. It doesn't hurt that there is no fat in grapefruit either—Susan can eat all she wants! And she doesn't even have to dig out the seeds. Grapefruit seeds, which so many people meticulously avoid, can and should be eaten. They contain powerful infection fighters. Grapefruits are also champion fruits when it comes to cardiovascular health. They protect your arteries and balance your blood cholesterol levels, benefits most likely due to their high fiber and high vitamin C content.

Would you believe that a kind of wonder fruit is currently being grown and brought to market that does several things for your health all at once? It's an excellent source of fiber—always important—but beyond that, it combats intestinal infections, inflammation, diarrhea, and overly acidic stomach. Over half of your immune system is associated with your gastrointestinal tract, so I always say that the road to health is paved with good intestines. This is one fruit that is excellent for good intestines.

The wonder fruit I'm talking about also excels at helping the body to detoxify and fight viral infections. It has been shown to lower blood cholesterol, lower blood pressure, and even stabilize blood sugar. Don't you want to consume this amazing fruit every day? There's a well-known saying that tells you that you should: "An apple a day keeps the doctor away." The wonder fruit is God's magnificent creation, the apple.

The only way to find out if that saying is true is to start eating an apple a day today. (I personally believe two apples a day can keep the doctor away for twice as long.) And as with the grapefruit, don't throw out the apple seeds—or the skin, or the core. Did you ever see a horse spit out any part of an apple? There's a reason why another saying goes "He's as healthy as a horse." Horses eat the whole apple, and so should you.

You may have heard that apple seeds are toxic, but don't worry. Although they do contain trace amounts of cyanide, your normal, healthy cells contain an enzyme that renders the cyanide inactive. Interestingly, cancer cells do not contain this important enzyme, so chewing apple seeds can actually help your body kill cancer cells while not harming normal cells. I call this God's chemotherapy!

> *...chewing apple seeds can actually help your body kill cancer cells while not harming normal cells. I call this God's chemotherapy!*

Go ahead, eat the whole apple—seeds, skin, core, and all. It will do you far more good than harm, and your fiber consumption will be off the charts.

Everything in Moderation

I t's simply not true that you must cover healthy foods in chocolate to make them palatable—though that works. But only in moderation. Everything in moderation, as the wise saying goes. Your perspective is what counts when it comes to foods like chocolate and other delicious but so-called "sinful" treats. Are they sinful or aren't they? Let's check the owner's manual on that. Proverbs 13:25 says, "The good man eats to live, while the evil man lives to eat" (TLB). Do you see a difference between the two?

Proverbs 13:25 says, "The good man eats to live, while the evil man lives to eat" (TLB).

Clearly we shouldn't be obsessed with food, especially unhealthy food that replaces good nutrition and robs us of good health.

On the other hand (and you chocoholics will be glad to know there's another hand), insisting that the only reason we eat is to fuel our bodies is like saying the only purpose for sex is procreation. Neither is true. God wants you to *enjoy* food (not to mention sex with your spouse). In the Bible, food is often linked with celebrations, and God's people are celebrant people. The Old and New Testaments are full of feasting—religious feasts, wedding feasts, and dinners for Jesus at rich tax collectors' houses.

Trust me, the people of the Bible ate more than leeks and onions. You can eat anything *in moderation.* As Philippians 4:5

Philippians 4:5 says, "Let your moderation be known unto all men" (KJV).

says, "Let your moderation be known unto all men" (KJV). Susan and I teach that the food choices that *typically* characterize you are what's important and that enjoying a (very) occasional delicious treat is not wrong.

Some people in our seminars see us as killjoys, and at break time or when we go out to eat with them, they are afraid to eat anything around us. If only they knew what happens on my birthdays! Every year, my mom makes her special recipe chocolate cupcakes for me, and though I am *typically* characterized by healthy food choices, when my birthday comes around, watch out!

Indulging in the occasional treat is not a problem. Indulging in a gluttonous lifestyle is the problem, which is why Proverbs 23:2 warns, "put a knife to your throat if you are given to gluttony" (NIV). Gluttony is a real issue for many people today, though most people don't even think about it in those terms. They think of it as being a "junk food junkie," and junkie is a more apt term than most of us realize. Americans don't die of old age anymore; they dig their own graves with a knife and fork and kill themselves with their own teeth. People who are quick to condemn alcoholism and illicit drug use don't even bat an eye as they, themselves, consume copious amounts of junk food.

Did you realize that the average American's food choices include an annual consumption of 750 donuts? That's more than 2 a day! Add to those donuts 60 pounds of cakes or cookies, 23 gallons of ice cream, 22 pounds of candy, 90 pounds of fat, and 365 soda pop servings. I guarantee you won't see numbers like that if you add up the average American's annual consumption of fruits and vegetables. We read in 1 Corinthians 6:19 that our bodies are the temples of the Holy Spirit, but if some of us don't change our food choices, we're going to change our temples into cathedrals!

If we go the world's way, we'll reap the world's results. Because of poor food choices—downright gluttonous food choices in many cases—the average American these days is both overweight and undernourished. That's amazing in the most agriculturally productive country in the history of the world. Every day here in the U.S., we produce enough food to feed ourselves—and we throw away enough food to feed another 50 million people! Yet the way we process most of that food robs it—and therefore us—

of almost any nutritional value.

I call it the "great nutrition robbery." We're robbing ourselves of the nutrition our bodies need and paying dearly for it in the process. "Why do you spend money for what is not bread, and your wages for what does not satisfy?" God asks in Isaiah 55:2. Another Scripture verse appropriately asks why we spend money

"Why do you spend money for what is not bread, and your wages for what does not satisfy?" God asks in Isaiah 55:2.

on "deceitful meat" (Proverbs 23:3, KJV). Why indeed spend our hard-earned money on "deceitful meat"? That *is* a good question!

God continues in that same verse, "Listen carefully to Me, and eat what is good, and let your soul delight itself in abundance." That's what we need to do, but our culture is going in the opposite direction. We process the good nutrition out of our foods, and along the way we add unhealthy and unnecessary calories as well. Besides huge amounts of excess sugar, our foods are also laced with man-made additives. Over 2,800 FDA-approved food additives are on the market—and on your pantry shelves if you're not careful while filling your grocery cart.

Our way of death is directly related to our way of life. My father consumed a huge number of unhealthy and unnecessary calories from junk food. At the age of fifty-six Dad weighed 289 pounds, and he blew out his aorta. God blessed him with a miracle—a skilled surgeon was able to repair it, and instead of needing the usual forty units of blood during the operation, Dad needed only two. Amazed, the non-Christian surgeon commented, "We got a heavenly consult on this one!"

Dad then got serious about doing the do's for a while and dropped down to 200 pounds, but his poor health habits still had a death grip on him. He soon skyrocketed back up to 289 pounds, and then it was too late. He couldn't ward off the terrible results of his self-neglect any longer, and his heart completely gave out.

Dad also loved caffeine. He drank a lot of coffee. Since he and Mom lived next door, I used to walk over, raid his cupboards, and take away his coffeepot. Susan can tell you how furious he got at me, but I wanted him around to see his grandchildren grow up! However, he only saw our sons—our daughters won't get to meet him until we join him in heaven. I know Dad is happy being with the Lord, but *we* miss him. Mom misses him, too. It's sad because it didn't have to be that way, but Dad was characterized by poor food choices that eventually killed him.

When I was younger, I certainly took after him. I'd wake up in the morning and toast my cinnamon toaster pastry. I'd load up the backside with butter and pour myself a glass of soda to go with it. (I needed caffeine, but I didn't like coffee.) That was "breakfast." For lunch I had my usual hamburger and fries. Thin as I was, unhealthy food was on my mind—and on my plate—all the time. It was fast, convenient, and it satisfied my unhealthy cravings. Susan was the same way. She became anemic back in high school because she didn't eat properly, and the more vitamin and mineral deficient she was, the more her palate craved the wrong foods.

Veterinarians call it pica when an animal has abnormal cravings for unhealthy substances. Some horses with pica start cribbing, or chewing on the wooden frames of their stalls. Obviously that's not good for them, nor does it solve their pica issues. It makes their health even worse.

As it is with some cycles we humans get into. For instance, large numbers of people go around and around in the chromium cycle. Chromium is an important trace mineral. You don't need a lot of it, but if you're not getting it, you're in a bad way. Chromium has many benefits. It builds muscle, helps burn fat, lowers cholesterol, and helps balance blood sugar and ward off mood fluctuations. When you lack chromium, you crave sweets. Yet if you eat sweets, they cause your body's chromium supply to be further depleted. The less chromium you get, the more you crave sweets, and the more sweets you eat, the less chromium you have.

It can be hard to get off that kind of merry-go-round, but until you give your body the nutritious foods it needs, you will suffer from such cycles. Pay attention to this verse of my "10 Keys" song and you'll do better.

> *Too much sugar will rob you*
> *Of minerals and vitamins.*
> *Sweet foods make fat—can you imagine that?*
> *So don't eat much of them!*

By the way, sweet foods do more than make fat and cause imbalances such as the chromium cycle. They also cause your moods to cycle, promoting unwelcome behaviors. You've probably heard that excess sugar causes hyperactivity in children. If you doubt it, consider the actual study done with several thousand prison inmates. The group was divided in half, and one half was fed a diet of nutritious, natural foods and beverages. The other half was fed a high-sugar, high-fat, low-fiber diet of processed foods and beverages. In the natural foods group, unruly and violent behaviors markedly *decreased*. In the other group, eating processed foods, the behaviors were horrible, even for such a prison setting.

Then the diets of the two groups were reversed—the healthy foods group was put on the unhealthy, processed foods, and the other group was put on the nutritious, natural foods. In a short period of time, the formerly well-behaved group became unruly and violent, whereas the out-of-control group, now on a diet of natural foods, became much calmer and less difficult.

The reason behind the results lies in the human brain's extreme sensitivity to any decrease in thiamin, or vitamin B1. The excess sugar in processed foods causes the brain's level of thiamin to greatly decrease, and as you might have guessed, the level of thiamin directly affects a person's inhibitory response to stimuli.

In other words, when your thiamin level drops, so does your

ability to say no to impulsive or improper behaviors. Without enough vitamin B1, the brain loses its ability to make certain inhibitory proteins, which are proteins that keep you from doing things you know you should not do. Simply put, you lose your inhibitions and poor behavior becomes the rule instead of the exception.

> *You increase not only your physical health, but also your mental and emotional health when you eat nutritious foods.*

As the study showed, poor decision making and poor behavior can be directly related to nutrition. You increase not only your physical health, but also your mental and emotional health when you eat nutritious foods.

Simple Yet Profound: How Susan Gets More Fruit into Our Day

Knowing you should get more fresh fruits into your daily diet is one thing. Making it happen is quite another. Our eating habits have been with us all of our lives and that makes them even harder to change. In addition, the busy schedules we keep make it really easy to fall into the junk food, fast food and convenience food trap. How can you keep bad habits and the time crunch from sabotaging your health?

Buy it.

Buy fresh fruits and vegetables so they are always on hand. Stock up with fresh apples, oranges, grapefruit and bananas. (Choose organic if you can!) These are available year 'round at your grocery store. Include blueberries, strawberries and melon in season. When you get home from the store, rinse, slice and store your fruit so it's easy to see and ready to eat. Set some out in a bowl on the table or counter to make them even more accessible.

Snack on it.

Now that you're stocked up on fresh fruits, clear out the junk food. Then, when the next snack attack hits you, you'll be more likely to grab a piece of fruit rather than a cookie, chips or some other over-processed, under-nourishing snack food.

Add it to water.

Lemons, limes and strawberries jazz up your glass of water, provide you fruit-nutrition and help you break the soda pop habit.

Cook with it.

Add fresh blueberries to oatmeal; top pancakes with strawberries and bananas or fill them with grated apple; add kiwi cubes, apple slices, grapes or dried cherries and cranberries to tossed salads.

Shake it up.

Add fresh or frozen berries to plain yogurt or a protein shake.

Bring it along.

When you leave the house, bring a little cooler of fruit along for the ride. Make fruit and veggies your first pick when packing lunches.

Midnight snack it.

Have fruit on hand for those nights when you wake up and can't get back to sleep. It's easier to digest and won't interfere with resuming a good night's sleep.

Key 7

Vegetables Keep You Fresh

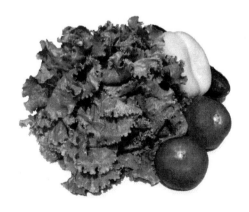

Broccoli, cabbage, and carrots
Will go to work for you;
They fight cancer and aging
And make you feel good too.

That's the verse I sing after the fruit verse. Vegetables are incredible! Jesus ate them. Some versions of Matthew 12:1 relate an incident where Jesus and His disciples were walking through a field of corn on the Sabbath and His disciples were hungry, so they began to pluck the ears of corn and eat them. (Other versions say the field contained grain or wheat, and those are healthy too. We'll get to them next.) Jesus and His followers thought eating raw corn was a good way to satisfy hunger, and they were right. You might think, *Raw corn? Who would eat that?* Yet raw corn is one of the healthiest foods for your gastrointestinal tract. Try it sometime.

We're raising our kids to follow Jesus in their eating habits. One day Susan took our hungry kids to the grocery store (always a mistake). In the produce section, one of them grabbed a cucumber and one of them grabbed an ear of corn, and they sat in the back of the grocery cart and ate their vegetables. Susan says it was cute, but funny because she was getting strange looks from people. The kids were getting strange looks, too, because they were obviously enjoying their vegetable choices.

We've found that the easiest way to get our family to eat vegetables every day is to make the veggies attractive and available. My mom is good at cutting up veggies and setting them out to for snacking. If you cut up some celery, carrots, cherry tomatoes, and even broccoli and cauliflower into small, snack-sized pieces, you'll be amazed at how fast those veggies will disappear from the tray you leave sitting out on your counter.

Susan likes to start the day with our kids by letting them make fruit and vegetable faces on paper plates. The faces change every day depending on what's in the refrigerator, and it's a great way to expose the kids to different foods. Cucumber eyes look great with carrot pupils, green or red peppers make perfect mouths, celery works well for ears, and an almond or walnut makes a nice nose. Don't forget to slice some fruit in thin strands or sticks for the hair!

Vegetables give you nutrients you can't get anywhere else. Did you know cabbage is the only known food source of vitamin Q? Did you even know about vitamin Q? Eat your cabbage and you'll get it. Cabbage, broccoli, carrots, brussels sprouts, and cauliflower are some of the cruciferous vegetables, which are major cancer fighters. They're full of vitamins A, C, and E, the trace mineral selenium, antioxidants, and antiaging nutrients. What a lineup! You can't win good health without them.

> *Vegetables give you nutrients you can't get anywhere else. Did you know cabbage is the only known food source of vitamin Q?*

When you compare the one-fourth of the U.S. population who eat the *fewest* fruits and vegetables to the one-fourth who eat the *most* fruits and vegetables, you'll find that the one-fourth who eat the fewest have double the cancer rate of those who eat the most. Double the cancer rate! That's a shocking statistic!

Which group would you prefer to be in? I don't know about you, but I know which group my family and I prefer to join. We're eating our fruits and vegetables every day. We enjoy them, and so will you with a little creativity and training of your palate. You'll be much healthier as a result, too.

Training Your Kids (and Yourself) to Eat Fruits and Veggies

"Train up a child in the way he should go," says Proverbs 22:6, "and when he is old he will not depart from it." Train your kids early to choose God-made foods–not man-made foods. When they are older, they'll be accustomed to making good food choices, and they'll have you to thank for their good health.

"Train up a child in the way he should go," says Proverbs 22:6, "and when he is old he will not depart from it."

In the Hebrew, "train up a child in the way he should go" literally means "touch the palate" of the child. Jewish mothers used to touch the upper roof of their children's mouths, their palates, with whatever foods they wanted their children to like. And the children did grow to like the foods mothers introduced that way. Wouldn't it be so much easier on you and me if we had been trained to go the way of healthy food choices early in our lives? Maintaining good health will be easier for our kids if we help them make healthy food choices while they are young!

Try resurrecting your appetite and helping your kids be healthy and wise by training your palates to like God-made foods. It won't take long. Since Isaiah 57:19 says God creates the fruit of our lips (and fruit is a good thing), add these words to your training program as a positive confession: "I am God's child, and I like God's foods. God's foods are good foods, so I like good foods." That's more of a faith confession for some of us than for others, but it's true. Repeating it can work wonders in resurrecting your appetite.

The Significance of Signatures

On my tape series "You Are What You Ate," I talk about the doctrine of signatures, a fascinating study all by itself (see www.drdonmd.com for ordering information). Signatures are features in the appearance of natural foods that indicate what part of the body the foods benefit. In other words, God designed foods resemble the part of the body they help.

> *Signatures are features in the appearance of natural foods that indicate what part of the body the foods benefit. In other words, God designed foods resemble the part of the body they help.*

Signatures are especially significant in regard to fruits and vegetables because the connections are so obvious. Cut a carrot in cross sections. What do you see? There's a little circle in the center of the carrot with striations going out from it in all directions. It's an orange eyeball, or at least an orange iris. Sure enough, carrots are loaded with vitamin A that's good for your eyes. Have you ever seen a rabbit wearing glasses? See, it works!

Cut a tomato in cross sections. See how it's made up of chambers inside, like the heart? Sure enough, tomatoes are heart smart. The same with apples—doesn't an apple look almost heart-shaped and heart-sized? Apples are heart smart too, along with strawberries, which are also heart-shaped. Grapes look a lot like red blood cells, and sure enough they are loaded with antioxidants.

The long, hollow tubes running the length of celery stalks resemble the veins and arteries in our circulatory system, so guess what celery is good for? Right, it keeps that circulatory system going. Do you know anyone with high blood pressure?

Tell them to eat celery. The medicinal effects of eating three celery sticks a day may surpass any high blood pressure medication on the market!

The doctrine of signatures also applies to other healthy foods. Walnuts and pecans with their fissured halves look kind of like your brain. You guessed it—nuts contain essential fatty acids that are healthy for the brain. We eat nuts every day for brain power.

Kidney beans are kidney-shaped, of course, and they add fiber to your diet and help with waste elimination. A quarter cup a day of almost any kind of beans could lower your cholesterol by 19 percent. Add three raw carrots a day to that (also tube shaped, like your blood vessels), and bad cholesterol goes down another 11 percent, for an amazing 30 percent reduction in bad cholesterol levels just from eating two vegetables!

Beans and bowel function go together, as most of us realize. At one church, I was teaching about normal bowel functions. I explained that the bowel is a temporary waste tank and that the average American walks around with two to ten extra meals in his or her abdomen because the colon is not cleansed, which means toxic waste sits much longer than it should in the body. I explained how important it is to have a bowel movement every day, and that increasing water and fiber intake help the bowel empty out more efficiently. The pastor mulled that over for a few seconds, then he jumped up and said to his congregation, "I think what Dr. Don is trying to tell us is that it's not what you don't do that counts, it's what you doo-doo!"

> *...the average American walks around with two to ten extra meals in his or her abdomen because the colon is not cleansed, which means toxic waste sits much longer than it should in the body.*

That's a little graphic, but basically correct. If you don't have a daily bowel movement, your detoxification system isn't working properly. The Chinese have known this for a long time. A doctor who trained in China told me that one solicitous greeting there is actually "Have you had your bowel movement today?"

I wouldn't try that one on the next person you greet, but it is true that daily bowel function is a vital indicator of good health. People who eat enough fruits, vegetables, and whole grains have an intestinal transit time of 24 hours or fewer—food enters their body and within 24 hours the waste from that food exits. That's a healthy pattern. Fiber, the major structural component of God-made foods, is the main component necessary for that kind of regularity.

People who eat a high-sugar, high-fat, low-fiber diet have an intestinal transit time of 7 *days*. That's unhealthy. And this may sound odd, but they also have bowel movements that sink to the bottom of the toilet bowl. "Sinkers" indicate an unhealthy diet. "Floaters" indicate a more nutritious diet. They contain adequate fiber, which is activated by adequate amounts of water to do its work in the intestines. People who take in enough fiber and water have bowel movements that are larger and less dense—so they float.

If you want to check your general intestinal health, eat some corn and then watch. It's embarrassing but important to see if you're getting enough fiber. Determine your transit time by eating some corn and watching how long it takes to work its way through your

> *Fiber detoxifies you, fills you up, not out, and acts as a broom in your body to sweep away the accumulation of bad fats and the toxins they contain.*

intestinal system. Then increase your fiber intake accordingly.

Fiber detoxifies you, fills you up, not out, and acts as a broom in your body to sweep away the accumulation of bad fats and the toxins they contain. Getting the fiber you need will change your life—and possibly your future. Illnesses such as colitis, diverticulosis, diverticulitis, and colon cancer are completely preventable—and in many cases completely reversible—with the proper attention to fiber and water intake.

Bring on Bob and Larry!

Fruits and veggies are amazingly healthy, yet 20 percent of Americans eat no vegetables and 40 percent eat no fruits. We're not even talking fresh produce here, we're talking *any* at all! Of the veggies Americans do consume, 25 percent are French fries—if you can call those veggies. I can't.

If you're a parent or Sunday school teacher, no doubt you're familiar with Bob the Tomato and Larry the Cucumber, stars of the famous *Veggie Tales* productions. The creators of Bob and Larry chose to name their production company Big Idea. In Big Idea's mission statement, under "What We Believe," they state, "The irresponsible use of popular media (TV, film, music, etc.) has had a profoundly negative impact on America's moral and spiritual health." One of their goals at Big Idea is to counteract that negative effect with something positive.

I'd like to second their belief statement in regard to physical health. I believe the irresponsible use of popular prepared foods has had a profoundly negative impact on America's physical health. I could fill more than one book with fire-and-brimstone preaching about the sad state of America's eating hab-

> *I believe the irresponsible use of popular prepared foods has had a profoundly negative impact on America's physical health.*

its—it's amazingly appropriate that the acronym for the standard American diet is SAD! However, as you know by now, I prefer the positive approach. The Big Idea approach. Look at the company's core purpose: "to markedly enhance the moral and spiritual fabric of our society through creative media. . . . The world is full of media companies that are out to make a buck. The world desperately needs a media company that is out to make a difference."

I second those statements, too, in the area of physical health. My purpose is to markedly enhance the physical condition of my fellow believers (and anyone else in our society who will listen) through creative teaching about biblical health, and my goal is to make a difference, not a buck.

Interestingly, Big Idea and I parallel each other not only in belief and purpose, but also in the method by which we accomplish our goals. Whether you need to get healthy spiritually or physically, bring on the tomato and cucumber! Fruits and vegetables make all the difference in the world (yes, the tomato is actually a fruit, but *Fruit Tales* is harder to say). Fruits and vegetables are Keys 6 and 7 in my 10 Keys that Cure.

Be Creative!

Yet you *can* train yourself and your kids to crave fresh fruits and veggies in place of sweet and salty man-made junk foods with no nutritive value. Use a little creativity. Cut up some of the fruits and vegetables we've mentioned and show your kids the significance of signatures. Tell them they're making their brains and eyes and hearts strong and healthy when they eat the foods designed to look like those parts of their bodies. Challenge them to examine natural foods and see if they can figure out what anatomical systems or organs they might benefit. Believe me, your kids will be fascinated, and they'll want to try new fruits and veggies more than ever before.

Another method is to arrange cut-up fruit and veggie pieces

attractively on a tray (eye appeal is buy appeal) and add a dish of healthy dip like vanilla yogurt for fruit or hummus (blended chickpeas) for vegetables. Or pop in a *Veggie Tales* video and let the kids eat tomatoes and cucumbers while they watch Bob and Larry. Make it your goal to eat two to three servings of fruit and five to seven servings of vegetables daily—at a minimum. As I said, Susan and I try to compose 50 percent of our family's diet from these power-packed foods. Put a little time and ingenuity into resurrecting your appetite and that of your family toward fruits and vegetables. It's time and effort well spent because it yields healthy results a hundredfold!

Simple Yet Profound: Resurrect Your Appetite

Sometimes eating healthy comes down to acquiring a taste for what's good for you. I promise this next statement is true, even though it sounds unbelievable: Your body *will* crave God-made foods that are good for you if you give it the chance. It's a matter of resurrecting your appetite.

Common sense says that since God wants us to live an abundant, joyful life and since He created certain foods to fuel our bodies, we should also be *designed* to enjoy those foods, right? And we are! It's just that some of our bodies have forgotten how to enjoy God-made foods because they are so overwhelmed with cravings for the wrong foods. Our bodies *will* crave whatever we feed them—which is why so many of us crave the wrong foods. We just need to feed our bodies the right things!

We all experience food cravings. How can we resurrect our appetites so our bodies crave God-made foods instead of man-made foods? Start with a little step of faith. We were invited to one church in New York to present our health seminar, and after Sunday morning service Susan and I went to lunch with the pastor and his wife. The pastor decided then and there to take a little step toward resurrecting his appetite. Our meal was buffet style, and Susan loaded her plate with carrots, cucumbers, and fruits—all healthy, God-made foods. The pastor looked at Susan's plate, looked at his own plate piled high with not-so-healthy choices, then looked back at Susan's plate again. I could see the wheels of his mind turning as he considered the material he had heard us present.

"Susan, can I see your plate a second?" he finally asked my wife.

"Sure you can," Susan responded, gracious but puzzled.

He moved his own plate to the side, grabbed Susan's plate, and placed it in front of himself. "How does that look?" he asked his wife. "Do you think I could get used to that?"

His wife laughed and shook her head a little at the unusual sight. At least he was experimenting to see how a plate of God-made food looked in place of his usual fare. Susan made him try a cucumber before he handed her plate back.

You may dislike certain foods right now—particularly certain fruits and vegetables—but if you know they're good for you and you start to eat them because you know it's the right thing to do, you will soon find yourself actually craving them. Amazingly, God designed you that way. He is the ultimate Engineer, and His work in designing your body and your appetite will pass the test. Try it!

A pastor at another church where we presented our seminar told us his story about going on the mission field. He was advised to eat plenty of yogurt before leaving because yogurt is filled with *Lactobacillus acidophilus*, "friendly" bacteria that promotes intestinal health. He was likely to encounter some unfriendly bacteria where he was headed, so he had to prepare ahead of time by giving his body the tools it needed to ward off illness.

"I never liked yogurt before the mission trip," he insisted. "I hated it so much that I had to plug my nose to eat it. Now I eat yogurt all the time, and I like it. I can't believe it!"

Granted, yogurt is not a fruit or vegetable such as we're talking about, but natural yogurt is wonderful food and this story illustrates my point—you *can* resurrect your healthy appetite.

Key 8

Bread from Heaven

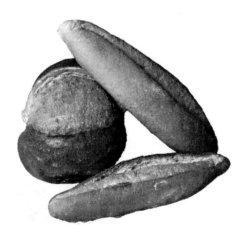

God once commanded the prophet Ezekiel to strikingly illustrate the siege of Jerusalem, and He gave Ezekiel specific instructions about how to do so. The prophet was to lie on his left side, bearing the sin of the House of Israel, for 390 days. During that time, he was to live on a set ration of bread and water. God didn't want His prophet to die during this time, so in Ezekiel 4:9 He gave the prophet a recipe for bread that would sustain life. "Take wheat, barley, beans, lentils, millet, and spelt, and put them into one vessel and make bread of them," God instructed. "According to the number of the days that you shall lie upon your side, 390 days you shall eat of it" (AMPLIFIED).

"Take wheat, barley, beans, lentils, millet, and spelt, and put them into one vessel and make bread of them," God instructed. " Ezekiel 4:9

Ezekiel bread sounds hearty, doesn't it? You could live on bread like that too. Have you tasted it? It's the best whole grain bread recipe ever, and it's right out of the Bible. Ezekiel bread's popularity is on the rise, and you can buy it under that name in many stores and bakeries now. Granted, the prophet Ezekiel may have tired of the taste after eating it day after day, but he lived on it *390 days* by God's command (along with water), so it really is food capable of sustaining life. And it's good.

> *God knew these foods would sustain His prophets' lives, and they'll sustain us as well.*

Whole grains in general are good. They are the undisputed kings of the fiber foods. One of the ingredients in Ezekiel bread is millet, which Susan loves. Millet alone can sustain life. If all you had was millet and water, you'd be all right. Not familiar with millet? Grab a handful of birdseed from your garage and take a look. Millet is the little, round grain in birdseed. But why throw all the good stuff to the birds? We ought to be eating millet too. In our house, we do eat birdseed every day—we buy breads, cereals, and pastas with millet in them.

Great, this doctor wants us to relax, breathe deeply, and eat birdseed, you may be thinking. I promise it beats the alternative—living stressed out, lacking fresh air and sunshine, and eating non-nutritious foods that sap your strength instead of supplying it. Even if it means eating birdseed now and again, doing the do's in my 10 Keys that Cure will bless and strengthen you!

In this chapter, let's take a closer look at the final three of the 10 Keys that Cure—whole grains and water, which Ezekiel lived on, and also what the Bible calls "clean" meats. God once told another prophet, Elijah, to go into hiding for protection, and God commanded ravens to feed him. Elijah "went and stayed by the Brook Cherith, which flows into the Jordan. The ravens brought him bread and meat in the morning, and bread and meat in the evening; and he drank from the brook" (1 Kings 17:5–6). That's another example of a prophet living on bread and water, this time with a little meat thrown in (actually, flown in). God knew these foods would sustain His prophets' lives, and they'll sustain us as well.

Whole Grains

Grains can be consumed in many forms, but when most of us think of grains, we think of bread. And when most of us think of bread, the first loaf that comes to mind is soft, white bread. Did you know white bread is the number one most frequently purchased item in the grocery store? That's because it's a staple of SAD, the standard American diet (and it *is* sad). It's not a staple at our house, though, and it shouldn't be at yours either. Why buy into SAD white bread when you can buy bread made with the good whole grains God created to really nourish us?

You may wonder, *Why grain bread? It's heavier and more*

expensive, and I can get white bread for less than a dollar a loaf at the bread store! That line of thinking brings me to the next verse of my song:

> *Please don't eat that white bread,*
> *The good nutrition's gone.*
> *Whole wheat, rye, and good brown bread*
> *Will make you big and strong.*

It's true whole grain breads tend to be a little heavier, but that's a good thing. Once you taste their flavor and realize how satisfying they are, you'll never go back! Again, it's a matter of training your palate to appreciate God-made foods, and they do make you feel healthier.

Why buy into SAD white bread when you can buy bread made with the good whole grains God created to really nourish us?

The only thing white bread makes you feel is a big mass of gluey glop in your stomach. Try this sometime: Put two pieces of soft, white bread in a bowl and add a little water. Stir it up. What does it remind you of? Right—glue. White bread is made from bleached or enriched flour—all the nutrition is gone, then sugar and loads of preservatives are added to keep that appealing but unhealthy loaf "fresh" on store shelves.

Did you know even rats, who will eat anything, can't survive on white bread? When scientists tried feeding laboratory rats exclusively on white bread, guess what happened? They proved there's truth in the saying "The whiter the bread, the sooner you're dead." The rats died—and it didn't' take long. There's nothing left in white bread to keep them alive.

Beware of anything that says *bleached* or *enriched* or *fortified*. Those words mean all the good, healthy fibers like grain husks have been removed from processed grains and fed to farm animals, who do all right while we eat the leftovers in the form of white bread and suffer ill health as a result. Did you know God indicated in Isaiah 28:28 that overprocessing grain damages it? "Grain for bread is crushed. Indeed, he [the farmer] does not continue to thresh it forever. Because the wheel of his cart and his horses eventually damage it,

> *God indicated in Isaiah 28:28 that overprocessing grain damages it? "Grain for bread is crushed. Indeed, he [the farmer] does not continue to thresh it forever.*

he does not thresh it any longer" (NASB). In other words, process grain too much and the good nutrition's gone!

Don't select white bread at the grocery; grab whole grain bread instead. A good rule of thumb when buying bread is that any loaf you can easily crush should be left at the store. Now, that doesn't mean you should visit the bread aisle and leave a trail of crumpled bread bags in your wake. (The store will kick you out in a hurry.) But give that loaf you're about to put into your cart a gentle squeeze. If you can't feel some solid texture between your fingertips, you know there's nothing in there to nourish and sustain you. It's not much more than air, sugar, and preservatives—in essence a dessert, and not a very good one either.

Whole grains are powerful health promoters. Ezekiel bread is a sprouted grain bread that even has some beans in it so it's high in fiber, which is great for your intestinal tract. That's important—I always say the road to health is paved with good intestines.

> *I always say the road to health is paved with good intestines.*

We talked earlier about how your colon must function well for you to stay healthy, and Ezekiel bread will help.

You can incorporate whole grains into your diet in many appetizing ways. Try wheat, barley, rye, millet, or oats for starters. When Susan cooks up oatmeal for breakfast and tops it with blueberries, a touch of real maple syrup, and a dash of cinnamon, she says the taste reminds her of blueberry pie. At lunchtime we might have a turkey sandwich on whole grain bread, and for dinner a bowl of barley soup really hits the spot. Whole grains are wholly good for your health!

Simple Yet Profound: Read the Label

Another good rule is to read the ingredients on the labels of bread and any other food. If you can't understand the label or if it lists man-made foods, not God-made foods, you're better off without it. Food ingredients are always listed in the order of amount; the most prominent ingredient comes first, then the next, and so on. If bleached or enriched flour is ingredient number one and sugar is number two, leave that loaf at the store. And if you can't even decipher some of the ingredients, consider it a *warning* label, not a food label—stop and drop that loaf, and roll your cart over to one with a label you can understand.

I make it my policy that if I can't understand an ingredient on a food label, I don't put it into my body! That's one way to preserve my life by avoiding preservatives. Consider this actual example: A sign on a vending machine at a zoo read, *"PLEASE* do not feed vending machine food to the animals—they might get sick and die!" Think about that next time your kids are in line at a vending machine full of over-processed, over-preserved foods. We know better than to feed such food to animals, but what about our kids and ourselves?

Key 9

White if You Choose Meat

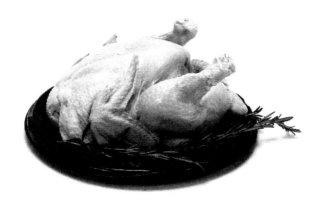

White bread is unhealthy, but white meat is just the opposite. If you choose to eat meat—and most of us do—then choose white. It's true that many people choose to be vegetarians rather than eating meat, and it's true that the Bible's first chapter designates fruits, vegetables, and whole grains as our food. It's also true that we were not originally designed to be meat eaters. Our intestinal tracts do most closely resemble that of herbivorous creatures, who have longer intestines with a low acid content. Carnivores, on the other hand, have shorter intestinal tracts and ten times the acid content. However, that doesn't mean the Bible insists that we eat an exclusively vegetarian diet. We've already seen that God commanded the ravens to bring Elijah bread *and* meat.

Consider also what God told Noah and his sons in the Bible's ninth chapter, after the flood: "All the wild animals, large and small, and all the birds and fish will be afraid of you. I have placed them in your power. I have given them to you for food, just as I have given you grain and vegetables" (Genesis 9:2–3, NLT). After Noah and his family disembarked from the ark, God added

I have given them to you for food, just as I have given you grain and vegetables" (Genesis 9:2–3, NLT).

meat to humankind's diet. He may have made this addition for a number of reasons. Presumably the flood would have destroyed all the edible vegetation, and it would have taken time for Noah and his family to plant and harvest crops. Perhaps they were in need of another source of nutrition. Whatever God's reasons, He told them they could eat meat, and the practice has continued ever since.

New Testament Scriptures also mention eating meat. Paul warns Timothy to watch out for those who command others "to abstain from meats, which God hath created to be received with thanksgiving . . . For every creature of God is good, and nothing to be refused, if it be received with thanksgiving: For it is sanctified by the word of God and prayer" (1 Timothy 4:3–5, KJV).

For every creature of God is good, and nothing to be refused, if it be received with thanksgiving: For it is sanctified by the word of God and prayer" (1 Timothy 4:3–5, KJV).

We can eat anything with prayer and thanksgiving, and it's right and good to pray over our food—especially some of the food we eat as part of the standard American diet. We better be praying over those food choices! I confess Mark 16:18 over my rare cups of coffee: "if they [believers] drink any deadly thing, it shall not hurt them" (KJV).

In the book of Leviticus, God distinguished clean from unclean meat choices and specified what the Israelites were to avoid. Even though today we are "not under law but under grace" (Romans 6:14), those Levitical laws are still important guidelines to eating healthy. Many Old Testament laws are still applicable today—even though we don't *have to* do them, we *get to* do them, and we want to do them because we know our Creator's wisdom goes far beyond our own.

Scientific research continues to prove the validity of many Old Testament laws dealing with health and nutrition. One amazing example is God's instruction to separate people who carried an infection. No one in Old Testament times knew about viruses and bacteria, yet God provided His people with laws that would prevent the spread of infection. Epidemics raged through Egypt and other ancient cultures, yet when the Israelites followed God's health instructions, they suffered none of those diseases.

The rest of us didn't catch on to the validity of some of the Old Testament's hygienic teachings until almost two hundred years ago, when Dr. Ignaz Semmelweis began to suspect that medical students with unwashed hands were passing horrible infections from bodies in the autopsy room to women in the maternity wards. In a Vienna hospital, Semmelweis sternly ordered medical staff to wash their hands in a chlorinated solution before examining women in labor. Immediately, the mortality rate of the mothers under his care dropped drastically.

Despite this astonishing result, Semmelweis was ridiculed for his beliefs. He was so maligned that he eventually left his position and committed suicide. Time and research have since proven the efficacy of his methods. Now that we can see through a microscope, we know why caution around infectious people makes good sense. Semmelweis was right all along—as was the Bible long before he came on the scene.

The same holds true with Old Testament laws regarding clean and unclean meats. God protected His people's health long before anyone understood the physiological reasons behind His rules. Even today it makes good health sense for many reasons to choose meats from the "clean" lists in the Old Testament and avoid unclean meats.

> *God protected His people's health long before anyone understood the physiological reasons behind His rules.*

Clean animals are those that chew the cud and have split hooves—sheep, oxen, deer, and the like. Unclean animals are the scavenger sorts—fish without fins and scales, certain birds, and pigs, for example. A whole Bible chapter, Leviticus 11, details clean and unclean meats. A widely known example from that chapter is that pigs are unclean (see verses 7–8). The Jewish people have always been well-known for avoiding pork, and I'm with them on that! Pigs eat anything and everything, so they accumulate astronomic levels of toxins in their tissues. Pork meat actually rots from the inside out, not the outside in—that alone ought to tell us pork is definitely not "the other white meat"!

As for sea creatures, Leviticus 11:9 tells us the healthiest to consume are those with fins and scales. Why are they clean? Fins and scales mean they're moving through the water, whereas creatures without fins and scales are probably bottom dwellers like lobsters (called the "cockroaches of the sea") and crabs. Bottom feeders filter the water, consume refuse, and accumulate toxins in their tissues, just as pigs consume trash with their land diet.

What about beef? An occasional meal of red meat is all right—lean, hormone-free beef can actually be healthier for you than cage-raised chicken with the skin left on. But beef still shouldn't be part of every main meal. If you were brought up on beef, as many of us were, try to limit your beef consumption to once a week. Once every two weeks is even better, and once you're used to that, try once a month. That may seem extreme in our beef-crazed culture, but when you're eating a healthy, tasty variety of other meats, you won't be asking "Where's the beef?" nearly as often as you think.

Limiting your overall consumption of meat and also dairy products is a good idea anyway. Believe it or not, 60 percent of all the antibiotics used in the United States are given to animals. That means when you eat a lot of meat and dairy products, you're getting way more than you bargained for.

> *60 percent of all the antibiotics used in the United States are given to animals. That means when you eat a lot of meat and dairy products, you're getting way more than you bargained for.*

Antibiotics and growth hormones pass along through the meat into you and your children, and too many antibiotics kill the good bacteria as well as the bad bacteria in your systems. You desperately need that good bacteria at work in you, and you need to replenish it by eating yogurt, apples, cabbage, figs, pineapples, and prunes.

You've probably also heard of people being immune to a lot of antibiotics, so their doctors have a hard time finding something to prescribe for them when they're ill. The cause isn't necessarily all the antibiotics they've been on in the past; it's all of the antibiotics they've indirectly been eating in animal products.

This doesn't mean you can never go to a wonderful seafood buffet, order a juicy beefsteak, or eat a fast-food cheeseburger. It means your diet shouldn't typically be characterized by such choices. Remember, God said to worship Him in spirit and in truth, not at the drive-up window booth!

Proverbs 23:20 tells us, "Be not among winebibbers; among riotous eaters of flesh" (KJV). If you're not among them, you won't be one of them! Who are "riotous eaters of flesh"? They

Proverbs 23:20 tells us, "Be not among winebibbers; among riotous eaters of flesh" (KJV).

are gluttons when it comes to eating meat. Most Americans fall into that category. The next verse goes on to say "the drunkard and the glutton will come to poverty, and drowsiness will clothe a man with rags" (NKJV). Ever feel drowsy after a huge meal, or after drinking alcohol if you've been down that road? It literally puts you in a stupor.

In the Bible, eating meat was connected to celebrations. People back then did not eat meat every day—and certainly not three times a day, as many of us do. Meat was saved for special occasions. The prodigal son's father, for example, gave instructions to "kill the calf we have been fattening" when his wayward son returned home. "We must celebrate with a feast" he said (Luke 15:23, NLT). The fatted calf was a treat, not an everyday meat!

It's best to moderate your meat consumption and learn the facts about the meats you eat. Do what Jesus did in John 21:12–14—eat the healthiest meat most often, clean fish. Jesus even thought fish were a good idea for breakfast. In one instance after

His resurrection, He appeared to some of His disciples who had been out fishing all night. They saw Him on the shore, and "As soon as they had come to land, they saw a fire of coals there, and fish laid on it, and bread. . . . Jesus said to them, 'Come and eat breakfast'" (John 21:9–12).

"As soon as they had come to land, they saw a fire of coals there, and fish laid on it, and bread. . . . Jesus said to them, 'Come and eat breakfast'" (John 21:9–12).

Jesus served His disciples the best of everything spiritually and physically. Fish is packed with nutrition and with the good fats and oils that lubricate your joints and boost your immune system and brain function. At our house we like fish, chicken, and turkey. They're lower in fat, and excess fat is where the toxins accumulate. For that reason, by the way, meat preparation is nearly as important as meat choice. If you leave on the skin, where most of the fat is, and fry the meat, you've greatly increased the fat content. Lean, skinless cuts are the way to go!

"All the fat is the LORD's," Leviticus 3:16 commanded the Israelites. (Wouldn't some of us like to make Him an offering of fat right now!) The next verse instructed, "This shall be a perpetual statute throughout your generations in all your dwellings: you shall eat neither fat nor blood." *Perpetual* means forever—in every generation, in every home, none of God's people were *ever to eat fat or blood*. With that strict perpetual command, the Lord was protecting His people's health. If you refrain from fat and blood, it will protect your health too!

Are Eggs Eggceptable?

While we're on the subject of protein-rich foods like meat, let's discuss eggs. In our presentations, the conversation always rolls around to eggs, and yes, the Bible mentions them.

Consider Luke 11:11–13:

> If a son asks for bread from any father among you, will he give him a stone? Or if he asks for a fish, will he give him a serpent instead of a fish? Or if he asks for an egg, will he offer him a scorpion? If you then, being evil, know how to give good gifts to your children, how much more will your heavenly Father give the Holy Spirit to those who ask Him!

This Scripture suggests to me that bread, fish, and eggs are *good* gifts (at least as opposed to stones, serpents, and scorpions). I agree. We've talked about bread and fish, and eggs are great too. Never mind the cholesterol—God put nutrients like lecithin into eggs to emulsify or help your body metabolize that cholesterol.

Eggs are also loaded with B vitamins and contain choline, which converts to acetylcholine in your body. That's the memory transmitter in your brain. You've heard that an apple a day keeps the doctor away and two apples keeps him away twice as long. I'd like to add that an egg a day helps your brain work the right way.

> *I'd like to add that an egg a day helps your brain work the right way. Eggs are a wonderful God-made food*

Eggs are a wonderful God-made food. Man cannot duplicate the egg—don't fall for those egg substitutes poured out of a carton. They're not much more than egg whites with artificial color added (and that's definitely not good for you). If you want to eat only egg whites, which are complete proteins by themselves, separate the yolks and throw them away. That's the inexpensive way to make egg substitutes—but why would you? I always eat both yolk and white. Yolks are loaded with good nutrition. God designed them that way. It's always best to eat God-made foods the way He made them, without processing them to death and taking out all the nutrients.

These divine principles of nutrition from both the Old and New Testaments still work in favor of your health today. So try some Ezekiel bread and other whole grain foods, eat an egg every day, consider fats an offering to God, skip the unclean meats, and choose white instead. Like the Israelites, you'll reap the benefits of biblical good health when you apply biblical nutritional principles to your food choices.

Simple Yet Profound: Get Hooked on Fish

If you're not a fish-eater, introducing fish into your daily diet can seem like quite a chore. My first advice is to choose fresh first, frozen second and use canned sparingly. The Old Testament dietary laws have good advice about which seafood to eat. The good fish are those that swim and have scales and fins, for example, salmon, tilapia, halibut, perch, orange roughy and tuna. These are clean fish that move through the water.

Crab, lobster and shrimp are bottom feeding scavengers that serve as the oceans' filters. The Old Testament actually prohibited eating them!

Two ways my family enjoys fish are when I broil it on tinfoil in the oven or sauté it in a little olive oil on the stove top. Squeezing a little lemon juice or topping with tomatoes during cooking can allay some of the fishy flavor.

Easy Oven Fried Fish

Change up this recipe with your favorite seasonings, herbs and spices.

- 2 lbs. Fish fillets
- 1 T. lemon juice
- ¼ fat free milk
- 2 T. hot pepper sauce
- 1 t. fresh minced garlic
- ¼. T. each, salt, pepper and onion powder
- ½ C. whole wheat bread crumbs
  (make them from the crust ends)
- 1 T. olive oil for greasing baking dish
- 1 fresh lemon, cut in wedges

1. Preheat oven to 475° F.

2. Wipe fillets with lemon juice and pat dry.

3. Combine milk, hot pepper sauce, and garlic.

4. Combine pepper, salt, and onion powder with cornflake crumbs and place on a plate.

5. Let fillets sit in milk briefly. Remove and coat fillets on both sides with seasoned crumbs. Let stand briefly until coating sticks to each side of fish.

6. Arrange on lightly oiled shallow baking dish.

7. Bake 20 minutes on middle rack without turning.

8. Cut into 6 pieces. Serve with fresh lemon.

Yield: 6 servings

Key 10

Drink What You're Mostly Made Of

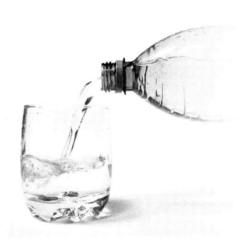

Y ou could say health starts with a five-letter word: *W-A-T-E-R*. Your body is mostly made of water. Between 65 and 70 percent of your body is water; your brain is more than 80 percent water, your blood is more than 90 percent water. Since your blood is mostly water and "the life of the flesh is in the blood" (Leviticus 17:11), you need water, water, and more water to be healthy.

"the life of the flesh is in the blood" (Leviticus 17:11)

You lose approximately 64 ounces of water a day from breathing, urination, and sweating, so you need to drink eight eight-ounce glasses of water just to break even and replenish yourself. Yet few people break even—most people drink much less. I cannot overestimate the number of people who walk around chronically dehydrated!

Do you often feel fatigued, irritable, depressed, confused, or beset by intense food cravings? You simply could be dehydrated. You can do a couple easy tests for dehydration. First, lightly pinch the skin on the back of your hand together and pull upward. If your skin doesn't immediately recede back into place when you let go, but rather stays raised for a few seconds, you need more water. Second, check the color of your urine. It should be light, not dark or even yellow. If your urine is colored, you need more water.

Dehydration creates a multitude of physical problems. It also gives illness and disease a chance to take hold. Many illnesses are exacerbated by or even result from chronic dehydration. Often, when the doctor diagnoses an illness, you're not so much sick as you are *thirsty*. You just don't know it. The medical community often ends up treating the effects of your pitifully low water intake with medication. However, many medications can be poisonous to your body and generate undesirable side effects, so you want to avoid them as much as possible. In large part you can accomplish that by drinking the water your body so desperately needs. A well-hydrated body is a healthy body.

If you drink significantly more water, your sensitivity to your body's need for water will also significantly increase. The more water you give your body, the more you'll know when you need it. That's a healthy cycle start.

As a doctor, if I were forced to pick only two ways to improve my health, I would choose increasing my intake of water and fiber. It's hard to believe what a difference those make. Remember, half the health equation is detoxification (the other half is balancing the immune system). Water is the ultimate detoxifier. An increase of only five glasses a day may cut the risk of colon cancer by 45 percent, bladder cancer by 50 percent, and breast cancer by 79 percent. Cancer can only develop in an acidic environment, and guess what dehydration does? It causes your body to be acidic. Many of us live right on the edge of acidity—a real risk to our health—but the more water we drink, the more balanced our pH levels will be.

> *Water is the ultimate detoxifier.*

Water also acts as a powerful cleanser to remove the plaque from artery walls, and it is instrumental in stabilizing blood pressure. Water lubricates the joints to prevent arthritis, and it diminishes headaches. Dehydration can cause all kinds of painful symptoms, but water can decrease them all—or even make them disappear. Here's another health equation:

More Water = Less Disease

I believe 50 percent of all our health problems would disappear if we drank enough water. That's why the "10 Keys" water verse goes,

Water cleans your body
Outside and within.
Eight glasses a day is the natural way
For cleansing to begin.

Notice eight glasses *begins* cleansing. You need more water than that, but the song was originally composed for children, who need a little less.

We talked earlier about the great health benefits of the bread recipe God gave the prophet Ezekiel, but God also commanded him to drink water. "You shall also drink water by measure, one-sixth of a hin; from time to time you shall drink," God instructed (a hin being about a gallon). Then there was Elijah, to whom the ravens brought meat. God commanded Elijah to "hide by the Brook Cherith, which flows into the Jordan. And it will be that you shall drink from the brook" (1 Kings 17:3). If God commanded

"hide by the Brook Cherith, which flows into the Jordan. And it will be that you shall drink from the brook" (1 Kings 17:3).

His prophets to drink water from time to time throughout the day, it's probably a good idea for you and me too!

How Much Water Do You Need?

Many people do not relish drinking water. If you are among them, take heart. Your appreciation for water will increase if you'll only start drinking it. Try adding a slice of lemon or lime, or cooling your water in summer and warming it in winter. Leave out the sugary powdered drink mixes, hot chocolate, or coffee, though. Those don't have the same good effects on your health as water—quite the opposite. We'll see

> *Divide your weight in pounds by 2 and drink that many ounces of water. If you weigh 150, divide by 2 and drink 75 ounces a day—about 10 cups.*

....

why shortly. First, here's a simple way to figure out how much water you need every day. Divide your weight in pounds by 2 and drink that many ounces of water. If you weigh 150, divide by 2 and drink 75 ounces a day—about 10 cups. That way at least you're replenishing what you're losing, and once you're used to that amount, drink some more!

I know some of you are thinking, *Wow, that's a lot of water—I'll be drowning in it!* It's not hard to drink all you need if you try these suggestions: Start your day with a glass or two as soon as you wake up .You'll soon get used to it and even miss it if you don't drink it! Then, drink a glass or two before meals, which helps fill your stomach so you can eat moderately and maintain your ideal weight. Take water along in the car and drink it at stoplights. Keep water on your desk at work. The more it's readily available, the more you'll drink. Before you know it, drinking water will be one of your healthiest habits, and you'll feel ten times better than you do right now.

What Kind of Water?

These days people often ask me, "What *kind* of water should I drink?" You'd think water is water, but not so anymore. There's tap water, bottled water, flavored water, reverse osmosis water, and purified water—the list goes on and on. Let's go down that list. The simple answer to "Should I drink tap water?" is a resounding "No!" At least not if you have another water source. If you don't have another source, then undoubtedly the health benefits of drinking even tap water with all the chemicals in it far outweigh the detriments of not drinking enough water. Drinking tap water is by far better than drinking no water at all.

However, the way tap water is processed in most municipalities leaves it full of chemicals such as chlorine and fluoride. Have you ever looked at your bathwater and noticed it was blue? Or taken a drink from your tap and thought *This tastes like the swimming pool water I swallowed by accident?* Take the hint—water that looks, smells, and tastes bad *is* bad. Besides, drinking water should make you want more, not make you grimace at every gulp.

As one alternative, bottled water is available almost everywhere now. You're better off choosing water in a plastic bottle than pop in a bottle or a can any day. However, getting attached to those plastic bottles of water isn't the best way to go, especially if you get into the habit of refilling the bottles over and over. Granted, you're making a well-intentioned effort to increase your water intake, but at the same time you increase your body's intake of the harmful chemicals that leach into the water from the plastic.

Reusing the bottles accelerates the leaching process. More chemicals leach into a beverage from a reused plastic bottle than from a new bottle! Drink bottled water when it's the best choice available, but save yourself a glass bottle of some sort to refill time and again.

Flavored waters are increasing in popularity, and their labels list water, 100 percent natural fruit flavors, and zero calories— but watch out. Most have artificial sweeteners like diet soft drinks, and those poison you. (We'll talk more about soft drinks

> *Flavored waters are increasing in popularity, and their labels list water, 100 percent natural fruit flavors, and zero calories—but watch out. Most have artificial sweeteners like diet soft drinks, and those poison you.*

shortly.) Some flavored waters are also carbonated. I'm not a big fan of carbonation because it acidifies your body, setting you up for all kinds of disease. If you crave strawberry-flavored water, instead of buying flavored water slice a *real* strawberry into a glass of water. You can't beat the real thing. Cucumber water is also delicious and refreshing, and almost any restaurant will serve you a slice of lemon or lime in your water if you request it. Make your own flavored waters with natural ingredients.

Overall, purified water is the best by far. We personally like reverse osmosis filtration or carbon filtration, and at times we even use steam distilled water. A reverse osmosis water system is an excellent investment in your health. Reverse osmosis is a safe, effective way to remove the most common toxins found in water.

The important thing, though, is to use some type of filtration for your water. If all you can afford is a twenty-dollar, sit-on-the-counter type water filter from the grocery store, buy it today. It will filter out 98 or 99 percent of all the impurities in your tap water and vastly improve the "taste" as well. One way or another, supply yourself and your family with a source of fresh, purified water.

Can Other Drinks Count as Water Intake?

What about all those other drinks in your fridge or pantry? Can they count as part of your water intake? Absolutely not. You want to avoid most other drinks that are part of SAD, the standard American diet. Nothing can take the place of water, and most other drinks out there do you far more harm than good. If you knew what happens inside you when you drink some of them, you'd want the containers labeled with a skull and crossbones!

> *Nothing can take the place of water, and most other drinks out there do you far more harm than good.*

How many coffee addicts do you know? It's one thing to get up and start the day with a favorite beverage (after you drink your water, of course); it's quite another to get up and get hit by a nagging headache because you haven't had your caffeine fix.

As if the caffeine addiction weren't bad enough, drinking coffee also causes an excessive loss of vital calcium through urination, and it increases the risk of cadmium toxicity. Cadmium is in both caffeinated and decaffeinated coffee and promotes cancerous cell changes. Natural alternatives to coffee are much safer. For an energy boost and focused thinking, try green tea, Ginkgo biloba, and ginseng drinks.

As far as your health is concerned, there's nothing soft about soft drinks. They're *hard* on your body! The excess sugar and phosphates cause calcium loss, and the sugar turns to fat and depletes your body of B vitamins. Sugar (in soft drinks or anything else) also depresses your immune system by lowering white blood cell activity. Ever wonder why there's a higher incidence of colds and flu during the holiday season? Maybe low resistance to holiday treats and low resistance to illnesses are related . . .

Soft drinks also knock your pH balance off, acidifying your body and promoting aging and free radical damage. The pH level of colas ranges between 2.7 and 3.4. Normal is 7.0. Think about this: If you drop a tooth into a cup of cola, that tooth will completely dissolve in 10 days! Trucks carrying colas are required to put "Highly Corrosive!" signs on their tanks. Do you want that kind of acid working its way through your body? You need to drink more than thirty-two glasses of pure water to undue the nasty effects of one soft drink! Are you willing to fill up that can or bottle thirty-two times with water and drink it all after you down that soft drink?

Diet soft drinks are no better—in fact, they're worse. Artificial sweeteners in diet drinks and other foods are highly toxic. Anytime those sweeteners get above 86 degrees—and your body temperature is normally 10 degrees hotter than that—they break down into three poisonous substances. One is methanol (metyl alcohol); toxic levels of that cause blindness. Another is formic acid; that's what poisonous insects inject into you. Why do it to yourself? The third is cancer-causing formaldehyde. Those aren't substances you want roving around inside you.

And forget losing any pounds—with consistent use, artificial sweeteners actually cause weight gain! Think it over. Diet soft drinks have been marketed for about thirty years now, and the average weight of people in our society has gone up, not down. Obviously, we're not getting any smaller, but we are, on the average, suffering from obesity and diseases such as diabetes much more frequently.

Finally, what about alcohol? Did you know the Bible specifically warns us thirty-eight times not to abuse alcohol? It's a poison that directly damages the brain, liver, pancreas, and small intestine. The danger of killing brain cells is self-explanatory. A damaged liver is prey to hepatitis and cirrhosis. Pancreas damage ushers in diabetes. Small intestine problems lead to poor absorption of all nutrients, especially fat soluble vitamins (A, D, E, and K), B vitamins, folic acid, and vitamin C. Many of these nutrients are meant to protect the body from free radical damage that promotes aging and aging-related diseases like heart disease, cancer, and arthritis, but they can't protect you if your body can't absorb them.

Alcohol increases free radical formation, which makes it a two-edged sword in favor of aging. Ever notice how alcohol drinkers often look much older than they are? Those who routinely consume alcohol suppress their immune systems and age themselves prematurely. In addition, just two or more drinks of alcoholic beverages a day increase a person's chances of developing tumor growths by an almost unbelievable 80 percent!

If alcohol is so bad for you, you're probably asking why, then, is it so widely known that drinking some red wine every day is supposed to be beneficial to your health. There's a nutritional reason behind that finding that has nothing to do with the wine. When red wine is made by crushing grapes, the grape skins and seeds are left in during the process. People today are, generally, so nutrient depleted that those who drink red wine actually benefit not from the wine itself, but from the nutrients in the grape skins and seeds. You can gain the same exact benefit from red or purple grape juice, so don't fall for the "red wine is good for you" slogan as an excuse to consume alcohol. There is no good reason to risk your health by consuming alcohol.

I should note that my family and I do enjoy some other healthy beverages in addition to water. There is even one drink I'll give you credit for toward your daily water consumption—green tea. You can drink four cups of green tea daily in place of four cups water. Personally I drink about six cups of green tea daily. Green tea is loaded with health benefits. Manufacturers are now cashing in on that discovery. You can buy green tea soaps, shampoos, and even green tea ice cream—though I wouldn't recommend that daily! Nor would I recommend buying the green tea in plastic bottles at the store. It's usually loaded with either sugar or artificial sweeteners and other unhealthy additives. Stick to real green tea you can brew yourself.

At our house, we also like herb teas and fresh vegetable or fruit juices (or sometimes bottled juices with no additives). Since our bodies are mostly water, though, we drink what we're mostly made of. As my song concludes, water makes your health complete!

You're Feeling Better Already

We've covered a lot of ground in the last few chapters (not to mention learning how to stay connected to the ground). We've explored all 10 of my Keys to Health, found them in the pages of Scripture, and illustrated how to apply them in everyday life. You've learned how to four-six it (Philippians 4:6) and cast all your cares on the Lord so you can relax. You've rediscovered the importance of a good night's rest (early to bed, early to rise . . .). You've faced that infamous "E" word, *exercise*, and seen how beneficial it is to incorporate a little walking into your lifestyle. You know that fresh air and sunshine are good for you; they brighten both your day and your attitude.

From a nutritional standpoint, you now know it's possible to resurrect your appetite for healthy, God-made foods. You can train your palate and your family's to enjoy fresh fruits and vegetables. You were designed to enjoy them! You can buy whole grain Ezekiel bread at the grocery store and throw in a little clean meat on the side. God said it's all to be enjoyed with thanksgiving. And you can drink, drink, drink water and learn to love it (while praying Mark 16:18, that no deadly drink will harm you, over some of your other beverage choices).

With all that simple, practical information at your fingertips, you must be feeling better already! I hope learning about my 10 Keys to Health has helped you. Even if you pick one key at a time and apply it, your health will take a turn for the better. Every believer can enjoy biblical good health. You've learned how through the pages of God's Word. His marvelous health plan *will* work for you.

In the next and final chapter, we'll look at some related health questions that always come up in my presentations. Do you wonder about when to see a doctor? How about the necessity of vitamins and other supplements? What about the cholesterol scare? And how can you check for yourself whether you are in good health? I'd like to address these and some other health questions before we're through. Your health is your choice, and I'd like to help you choose the good life!

Simple Yet Profound: Sing a Little Song.

My mother, a retired schoolteacher, once had a classroom full of busy second-graders to whom she imparted her vast wisdom—when she wasn't drilling it into me at home. In her classroom I found my first platform for preaching about biblical health. Mom and my sister, who was also a second-grade teacher, invited me to come in on career day and talk to the kids about my medical profession and about health. As I attempted to distill my medical and scriptural knowledge about good health principles into a format second-graders could understand, the Lord helped simplify and clarify it in my mind. I ended up composing a little song that says it all.

That was more than twenty years ago, and it hasn't changed since. I'm still singing the same tune. Its chorus condenses my twenty-one years of school and twenty years of Bible study into a few simple lines. I wish I could share the melody with you through the pages of this book—once a child hears the catchy tune, they rarely forget it. Parents and grandparents who have bought our little CD will attest that once children learn the song, adults can't get away with anything! I will share the chorus with you here:

Dr. Don's 10 Keys that Cure

Learn to relax,
Get to bed on time,
And do your exercise.
Breathe fresh air
While the sun's out there,
And eat like this little rhyme:

Fruits and vegetables,
Whole grains,
White if you choose meat.
Drink what you're mostly made of,
Water makes your health complete.

My little song contains more verses that elaborate on these 10 keys, and we'll look at those as we go along. In a nutshell, though, if you do the do's in this song's chorus, you'll enjoy great health. You'll have all the energy you need to do the things God wants you to do.

Your Health Is Your Choice

Choose Life!

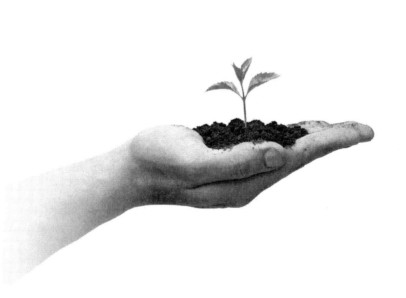

God told His people, Israel, "Today I have given you the choice between life and death, between blessings and curses. I call on heaven and earth to witness the choice you make. Oh, that you would choose life, that you and your descendants might live!" (Deuteronomy 30:19, NLT).

Oh, that you would choose life, that you and your descendants might live!" (Deuteronomy 30:19, NLT).

God presents His people, including you and me, with a multiple choice test here. We can choose A, life and blessings, or B, death and curses. Then God tells us the answer to the test— He says, "Choose life!" It doesn't get any clearer than that. God gives us the choices and tells us what to choose to enjoy life.

Notice, however, who it is who must choose. God doesn't choose for us. He has given every person a free will, and He always respects that. Each of us must choose to live for God or for the devil, to eat for good health or for poor health, to go the easy way or go the way of the transgressor, which is hard.

The devil cannot choose for us either. He'd certainly like to choose death for us, but he must also respect our God-given free will. The devil can't kill us, or we'd already be dead! If he could put into action a 5-minute plan that would take us out, he wouldn't hesitate another instant. He knows he can't do that, though, so what he does instead is attempt to deceive us into choosing what seems like a not-so-harmful road—a little sugar here, a little fat there, some highly processed, nutrient depleted foods, not much fiber or water in our diets. The devil wants us to typically make poor food choices, and day after day he whispers to us that the little choices aren't a big a deal. But beware, "There is a way that seems right to a man, but in the end it leads to death" (Proverbs 16:25, NIV).

If the devil can get us to choose death one day at a time—one bite at a time—he knows that eventually, even if it takes years, we'll destroy ourselves. He'll take advantage of us if we are ignorant of his schemes (see 2 Corinthians 2:11), but if we realize what he's up to, we can avoid his deadly detours and choose to stay on God's road to good health.

When we stick to God's ways and eat God-made foods, we reap the benefits God promises in His Word. Psalm 103:5 says it is the Lord who "satisfies your mouth with good things, so that your youth is renewed like the eagle's." Susan likes that thought—eat God-made "good things" and you'll look and feel younger!

Exodus 23:25–26 promises, "So you shall serve the LORD your God, and He will bless your bread and water. And I will take sickness away from the midst of you. No one shall suffer miscarriage or be barren in your land; I will fulfill the number of your days." Our family uses the beginning of this verse as our

Exodus 23:25–26 promises, "So you shall serve the LORD your God, and He will bless your bread and water. And I will take sickness away from the midst of you.

prayer before every meal: "Thank You, Lord, for blessing our bread and water and taking sickness and disease from the midst of us. In Jesus' name, Amen." We love its promises.

What blessings God pours out on us when we serve Him and live His way in every area of life, including nutrition! He says He will bless the food we eat, take away sickness and disease, bless the women in their childbearing, and insure that we live long lives. That's the best health-care benefit package you'll ever find!

What about Seeing a Doctor?

As we travel and teach, many people ask, "What about seeing a doctor? Does doing the do's and eating God-made foods mean I'll never have to go to a physician?" Not necessarily. I'm trained as a physician. Luke, who wrote the Gospel of Luke and the book of Acts, was called "the beloved physician" (Colossians 4:14). We call Jesus the Great Physician who heals all our diseases spirit, soul, and body. Jesus even talked about seeing doctors when He said, "It is not those who are healthy who need a physician, but those who are sick" (Luke 5:31, AMPLIFIED).

> *We call Jesus the Great Physician who heals all our diseases spirit, soul, and body.*

Seeing a doctor regarding a health question or concern is not a sin, nor does it necessarily show a lack of faith, but let me say this: The first doctor you should visit with your health issue is Dr. Jesus. You wouldn't believe the number of people who approach me about a health issue and stammer "Uh, no, not really . . ." when I ask "Have you prayed about your situation?" Most people can't give me a single Scripture either when I ask, "What verse are you standing on from God's Word about this issue?" Approaching the Great Physician is often the last thing that comes to people's minds—the last resort, the desperate measure, so to speak—when it ought to be the very first thing they do!

Three other doctors I recommend that you visit regularly are Dr. Diet, Dr. Quiet, and Dr. Merryman. Dr. Diet will tell you to eat the foods God created because "you are what you ate!" Your body is constantly changing—literally making itself new out of the foods you've eaten. For instance, every twenty-eight to forty-five days you have a brand-new skin. Your body "sheds" an astonishing forty pounds of dust over your lifetime in the form of skin particles (yes, dander or dandruff) as your skin becomes new. Every six weeks you have a brand-new liver, and it only takes three to five days for your stomach lining to be made new (because of the high acid content, the cells are exchanged quickly). In a twelve-month period, 98 percent of your atoms and molecules are replaced, all manufactured from the foods you consume. Do you want to be made out of a cream puff or a Hostess Sno Ball with no substance? Or do you want your body to be made of healthy, fresh, whole foods? You are what you ate!

Dr. Quiet will tell you to relax the way God both modeled and instructed when He instituted a Sabbath day of rest. The Bible promises, "A calm and undisturbed mind and heart are the life and health of the body (Proverbs 14:30, AMPLIFIED). That's

"A calm and undisturbed mind and heart are the life and health of the body (Proverbs 14:30).

my favorite health verse in all of Scripture (of course, I have many favorite health verses . . .). It's healthy to stay calm and relaxed. Practice more than stress management—practice stress elimination by four-sixing it and casting all your cares on the One who cares for you. And get the rest and exercise you need to rejuvenate body, soul, and spirit, as Jesus did.

Dr. Merryman will quote you Proverbs 17:22, "A merry heart does good, like medicine." Likewise, Proverbs 15:30 says, "A cheerful look brings joy to the heart, and good news gives health to the bones." Put simply, happier people are healthier people. I'm sure that's one reason the apostle Paul advised, "Friends, I'd say you'll do best by filling your minds and meditating on things true, noble, reputable, authentic, compelling, gracious—the best, not the worst; the beautiful, not the ugly; things to praise, not things to curse" (Philippians 4:8, MESSAGE).

"Friends, I'd say you'll do best by filling your minds and meditating on things true, noble, reputable, authentic, compelling, gracious... (Philippians 4:8)

On the other hand, Proverbs 14:30 warns us that "envy, jealousy, and wrath are like rottenness of the bones" (AMPLIFIED). Another version, the NLT, actually translates *rottenness* as *cancer*. That's too high a price to pay for harboring negative emotions. Get rid of any junk in your trunk like negative emotions, anger, unforgiveness, and anxiety. Trust in God's promise of an abundant life, and as Paul emphasized by saying it again and again, "Rejoice in the Lord always. Again I will say, rejoice!" (Philippians 4:4).

As for other doctors, there are appropriate times to pay them a visit. If someone in your family requires a couple stitches, for example, you probably don't want to handle that at home. And think about it—Proverbs says a merry heart does good *like a medicine*. That implies that medicine does some good.

I prefer, though, to use medicine in the form of natural remedies, which are safer than manufactured drugs. Many drugs manufactured today can be poisonous to your body and have nasty side effects. It's wise to find a physician who is judicious in what he or she prescribes. You also want to choose a physician who emphasizes nutrition and living a healthy lifestyle, not someone who concentrates on treating what ails you after the fact. Any good physician knows how true it is that an ounce of prevention is worth a pound of cure.

Doctors and medicines are sometimes a huge blessing. When you or someone you love suffers a traumatic injury or is involved in an accident, you better believe you want a skilled physician on duty in the emergency room! Where day-to-day health is involved, however, you'll want to apply the words of Hippocrates, the Greek physician considered the father of modern medicine: "Let your food be your medicine and your medicine be your food."

That's the whole idea behind God-made foods. The Lord "satisfies your mouth with good things, so that your youth is renewed like the eagle's" (Psalm 103:5). You'll live longer, look

The Lord "satisfies your mouth with good things, so that your youth is renewed like the eagle's" (Psalm 103:5).

younger, and need less medical attention if you'll do the do's and live according to God's perfect health plan.

To Supplement or Not to Supplement?

Many people ask me if it's still necessary to take supplements if they eat a balanced diet full of God-made foods. Just to keep from being deficient in the major vitamins and minerals, you'd need to eat two to four fruit servings, four to six vegetable servings, and five to eleven whole grain servings 365 days a year.

That's not very likely for most people, and it also presumes these fruits, vegetables, and whole grains are grown on nondepleted soils, which are difficult to find. United States Senate Document 264 tells us that over 90 percent of Americans are deficient in one or more minerals because of the depleted condition of our soil. Yes, taking supplements is a necessity for good health.

What supplements should you take? At a minimum, take a good multivitamin and some essential fatty acids, which I talk about in the section that follows on cholesterol. (For more specific information on supplements, visit www.drdonhealth.com.)

What about Cholesterol?

Cholesterol-managing drugs are the top-selling pharmaceuticals in this country. However, they can be as harmful as they are beneficial, depleting the body of essential nutrients. If that's the case, then what do you do about troublesome cholesterol levels? As with any medical problem, an ounce of prevention here truly is worth a pound of cure.

First, prevent cholesterol troubles by eating nutritiously and judiciously. I mentioned earlier that a quarter cup kidney beans and three raw carrots a day can lower bad cholesterol levels by as much as 30 percent. If you're on cholesterol medication, add those to your daily diet and next time your levels are checked, your doctor may reduce your medicine dosage or even eliminate it. If you really want quick results, add sweet potatoes to your diet too. They are the very best cholesterol-lowering food you can eat. Oats and garlic can also help lower your cholesterol.

Keep in mind, too, that eliminating every trace of fat from your diet is not the answer to your cholesterol troubles. You need to understand that there are good fats and bad fats. Knowing which is which is vital to good health. Toxins hide in bad fats, whereas good fats benefit the body. Every cell of your body needs to take good nutrition in and get waste out. Surrounding each cell—all 100 trillion of them—is a bilipid layer where fats can be stored. Bad fats, which are saturated fats derived mostly from animal products, gum up your cell membranes, that bilipid layer. Your cells can't work as efficiently.

Those bad fats heighten your LDL or "bad cholesterol" level and cause plaque on your arterial walls. Partially hydrogenated fats are horrible for your health, probably worse than anything else! Cakes, cookies, pies, and fried foods are loaded with them. And man-made trans fats, the kind where oil is heated and changed to make foods thicker and creamier, are horrible for you too. Margarine, for example, contains trans fat. Studies have concluded that thirty thousand Americans a year die as a result of a high-fat diet. It's no wonder in Leviticus 3:17 that God commanded the Israelites to eat no fat!

> *Studies have concluded that thirty thousand Americans a year die as a result of a high-fat diet.*

Bad fats cause every cell in your body to need an "oil change." Try a new oil, good fats. Make sure you get enough essential fatty acids, or "EFAs" as they are called in supplement form, to keep your cells properly lubricated. EFAs are good for your heart, your brain, your immune system—every part of you. They soften your skin, boost your energy level, and help you think clearly. Taking in the proper amounts of EFAs is essential to managing your cholesterol levels.

Nuts and seeds are great sources of EFAs, and so are oils such as olive oil and flaxseed oil. Fish is power-packed with them—that's why two servings of fish a week can lower heart disease by 40 percent. EFAs can also be taken in supplement form. I use flaxseed daily, as well as fish oils, to make sure I'm "changing my oil."

When it comes to cholesterol management, do the do's. Eat vegetables shown to greatly reduce cholesterol, avoid processed foods high in trans and partially hydrogenated fats, eat foods high in good fats, and supplement EFAs as needed. When you do the do's, you can escape the bad cholesterol trap!

A Self-Check Health Check

Here's a little health check for you that you can do yourself. Answer these questions truthfully:

1. Do you always handle stressors properly? Do you know how to four-six it?
2. Do you always get enough sleep? Are you asleep between 10 p.m. and 2 a.m.?
3. Do you follow a consistent exercise program? ("Yes" means you *are* following it, not you *plan* to follow it!)
4. Do you regularly get some fresh air and make a habit of deep breathing? Do you avoid smoking?
5. Do you regularly get some sunshine, daily if possible?
6. Are fresh fruits on your menu every day?
7. Are fresh vegetables on your menu every day? (French fries don't count!)
8. Are whole grains a main staple of your diet? Do you typically avoid SAD—the standard American diet of processed foods?
9. When you have a choice, do you choose white meat over other meats? Do you keep it lean?

10. Do you drink what you're mostly made of, water, at a rate of eight to twelve cups a day? Do you avoid alcohol, soft drinks, coffee, and other unhealthy beverages?

Did you notice that this list of questions is more like a pop quiz on my 10 Keys that Cure? How did you do? If you scored 10 out of 10, answering "Yes" every time, congratulations! Wonderful! You're either very healthy or soon to be that way.

If you could not answer "Yes" to each question, though, take heart. You can start putting into practice my 10 Keys that Cure immediately. Start planting the seeds of better health habits in your life today. Retakes of this health quiz are offered daily, so you can take it again tomorrow and do better than you did today!

Reaping "Life Abundant" in Your Health

Yance ou reap what you sow, so they say. That's true because it comes straight from the pages of Scripture: "whatever a man sows, that he will also reap" (Galatians 6:7). And nowhere is it

"whatever a man sows, that he will also reap" (Galatians 6:7).

more true than in the area of your health. I hope you have realized while reading this book that no matter where your current level of health is, you can do simple, positive things every day to reap the good health promised in God's Word. Don't hang a long list of don'ts on your refrigerator and pull a long face every time you look at them (or try *not* to look at them). It can be discouraging to keep thinking about how far you have to go and about all the things you will have to deny yourself to get there.

Instead, hang up my 10 Keys song lyrics and concentrate on the ten good things you can do that will help you gain ground health-wise every day. Be encouraged and smile when you think of how you *get to* do healthy things instead of *having to* do them. Thank God every morning for the energy to get up and get moving. If your health isn't good yet, thank God that you can at least move your big toe and do that much until you can do more!

Four-six it whenever a problem or worry comes to mind, casting all your cares on the Lord because He cares for you. Remember that God isn't in the business of de-stressing, He's in the business of no stressing. He intends your days to be a taste of heaven on earth, to be enjoyed, not endured. Get outside a little bit every day and take advantage of the fresh air and sunshine He created to give you both good health and pleasure.

Eat the foods God made for you, foods that fill and nourish you to keep you healthy and strong so you can accomplish everything He has purposed for you. Make fruits and vegetables straight from the ground 50 percent of your diet. Eat satisfying, high-fiber whole grains, try a loaf of Ezekiel bread, and avoid processed foods. Choose white meat, avoid fat, and limit your consumption of other meat products or "unclean" meats, knowing God handed down the concept of clean and unclean meats in Scripture to promote great health among His people. And of course, drink what you're mostly made of—water, water, and more water. Water makes your health complete.

Finally, stay in God's Word daily. God's Word tells us that He desires "that you may prosper in all things and be in health, just as your soul prospers" (3 John 2). When your mind (your soul) is renewed by the Word of God, you'll be transformed (see Rom 12:2), and you'll have the mind of Christ in regard to your health. You'll know what God's Word says about your health, you'll think healthy thoughts, you'll do healthy things, and you'll *be* healthy—for whatever a person thinks on in his or

> *When you follow God's plan in His Word, you'll reap "life abundant" in your health—body, soul, and spirit.*

her heart, he or she becomes (see Proverbs 23:7).

As John 10:10 assures us, Jesus came to give you and me life abundant. When you follow God's plan in His Word, you'll reap "life abundant" in your health—body, soul, and spirit.

One More Kind of Water

I want to suggest one more kind of water to you before we're through. "Those who drink the water I give," Jesus said to the woman at the well, "will never be thirsty again. It becomes a fresh, bubbling spring within them, giving them eternal life" (John 4:14, AMPLIFIED).

If you feel a thirsting inside you that's not physical, an intense longing for something more to life, though you're not quite sure what, you might be spiritually dehydrated. You need a drink of the Living Water Jesus was talking about. A relationship with God, your heavenly Father, your Creator, will satisfy your intense thirst deep down inside. If you don't know Him yet, you can come into His family right now by accepting His Son, Jesus, as your Lord and Savior. The Bible promises that "whosoever shall call upon the name of the Lord shall be saved" (Romans 10:13, KJV). That "whosoever" means *you*, no matter who you are, where you've been, or what you've done. If anyone, including *you*, will "confess with your mouth the Lord Jesus and believe in your heart that God has raised Him from the dead, you will be saved" (Romans 10:9).

Simply pray the following prayer out loud with all your heart: "O God, I come to You in Jesus' name. I believe that Jesus died on the cross, shed His blood for me, and paid for my sins. I believe He rose again and gave me the gift of eternal life, and I receive Him as Lord of my life. Jesus, I am Yours now and forever. I know You have a plan and a purpose for my life, and I believe You want me healthy and whole, spirit, soul, and body, so that I can serve You all my days. I thank You for giving me the Living

Water, and for hearing my prayer. I give you my life from this day forward. In Jesus' name, Amen."

Welcome to the family of God and to the river of life and health you'll find in knowing Him! The Bible promises that "His divine power has given to us all things that pertain to life and godliness, through the knowledge of Him who called us by glory and virtue" (2 Peter 1:3). Enjoying good biblical health certainly pertains to life and godliness! With that precious promise in mind, let's go out and live for God in great biblical health, blessing others as He has blessed us all along the way.

> *Welcome to the family of God and to the river of life and health you'll find in knowing Him!*

Dr. Don's
Easy Reference Guide for
Common Health Problems

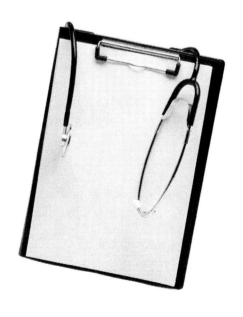

Dr. Don's Easy Reference Guide
for Common Health Problems

1

Achieving Ideal Weight: LEAN on the Lord

Do you want to lose weight? LEAN on the Lord. Don't skip meals. Instead, show your gratitude for the nourishment He provides by eating slowly and appreciating each bite. Did you know it takes your stomach 20 minutes to tell your brain you are full?

Eat only when you are hungry—physically hungry. Avoid the temptation to use food as a treatment for depression, anxiety or stress.

L - Liquids

Drinking plenty of water is important to good health and essential if you want to lose weight. Water constitutes up to 70% of your body tissues, 80% of your brain tissues and 90% of your blood. It detoxifies you, cleanses you and lubricates your very cells. If you want to lose weight, drink 8 to 12 glasses a day.

Start your day with water. Drink a full glass an hour before meals. Feeling hungry? Maybe you're thirsty! Fill up on a glass of no-calorie water and see if you can wait a bit longer before eating.

E - Exercise

Exercise does more than burn fat and calories. It gives you more energy and releases endorphins—those feel-good brain chemicals. Exercise also increases the oxygen-carrying capacity of cells throughout your body, boosting your immune system while building your muscle. Muscle is your best friend in weight loss. Try to engage in light exercise after meals to boost your metabolism.

Make a decision to start exercising NOW—even if you are relaxing in your recliner.

A – Add and Avoid
- Add high fiber, complex carbohydrate foods such as raw fruits, raw vegetables, and 100% whole grain breads and pastas.
- Add good proteins: legumes, egg white, lean meats and grilled fish.
- Add more fresh foods, prepared from scratch.
- Avoid trans-fats, saturated fats, hydrogenated oils and fractionated oils. These build fat that your body doesn't know how to burn.
- Avoid sugar, especially high fructose corn syrup—a highly processed monster that builds stubborn belly fat.
- Avoid fast foods and convenience foods that serve up bad fats, sugar and additives instead of God-given natural nutrients.

N – Nutrients
You're working hard, drinking water, eating right, exercising—so give yourself a boost! Add a good multivitamin with B vitamins, chromium and vanadium.

2
ADHD: Diet or Drugs?

Are you or your child...
- Hyperactive, fidgety and unable to sit still?
- Impulsive and unable to finish what you started?
- Unable to pay attention, making careless mistakes?

If you are human, you probably can answer "yes" to all of these, depending on what's going on in your life at the moment.

Or, you may be diagnosed with ADHD—a non-disease created to describe symptoms that could indicate food allergies, an over-stressed lifestyle, anxiety, depression, lead poisoning or some other learning disability.

I define ADHD as simple incompatibility between a person and their environment. Lifestyle changes can often solve the problem: change jobs, find alternative education, or improve your diet.

Eat real, not processed: fresh fruits and vegetables, whole grains and "brain" foods. Include flax seed oil for EFAs and fish oil or wild caught fish for DHAs and EPAs. Support serotonin production with turkey, sunflower seeds, and bananas.

Use the Pulse Test or an elimination diet rule out food allergies. Common triggers are sugar, cow's milk, wheat, yeast, corn, eggs and chocolate.

Supplement with a high quality multi-vitamin/mineral (B vitamins, calcium, zinc, magnesium and chromium are essential) and a glyconutrient source.

Detoxify. This high fiber diet and supplements will start the process. Reinforce with fasting and parasite control, if needed. Avoid toxins such as artificial colors, flavors, additives, preservatives—cook from scratch! Be aware that poor dietary absorption of naturally chelating nutrients can cause heavy metal toxicity.

Avoid chemical treatments. On February 9, 2006, a FDA advisory panel voted to recommend adding its strongest warning label—a "black box" label--for Ritalin, Adderall, Focalin, Methylin, Metadate, Concerta and other medications used to treat ADHD/ADD.

Start your day with a "Brain Shake."
- 1 scoop of soy protein powder
- 1 scoop of green powder
- 2 T. ground flaxseed
- 1 banana

- ½ C. soy milk
- ½ C. orange juice (not from concentrate)

Blend and enjoy a brain happy day!

③

Alkalize Your Diet and Kiss the Fat Goodbye

Do you know your pH?

Probably not. Chances are, if you eat like most Americans, your pH level errs on the acid side. Processed foods, fast foods and packaged foods all contribute to acidifying your body chemistry. Even naturally alkaline foods become acidic during industrialized food processing. Other acidifying agents are caffeine, alcohol and antibiotics. Stress and inactivity also cause acidity to rise.

An acid body environment causes all kinds of mischief, including weight gain and obesity. You see, the body responds to acidic molecules by wrapping them in tough-to-lose fat. It then stores them safely away from the heart—on the buttocks, abdomen and thighs. Acidic pH also causes blood sugar to rise. And that can be another factor in weight gain.

Eat Slimming Alkaline Foods!

Most fruits and vegetables, especially greens, are alkaline. Exceptions are cranberries and beans. You may wonder how acidic citrus fruits can be considered alkaline. The process of digestion actually turns them alkaline in your body.

Very High Alkaline Foods

- Bananas
- Chocolate
- Figs

- Orange juice
- Potatoes
- Spinach
- Watermelon
- Dandelion Greens
- Avoid Processed Foods!

Just because a food naturally is highly acidic does not mean it is unhealthy for you. Including naturally acidic foods in fresh, made-from-scratch recipes probably won't hurt you a bit. The problems, like weight gain, arise when your diet does not include alkaline foods but instead relies on processed, packaged and fast foods. You see, processing turns naturally alkaline foods acidic.

How Processed Acid Foods Impact Your pH

Human blood pH should be slightly alkaline (7.35 - 7.45). Below or above this range means symptoms and disease. If blood pH moves below 6.8 or above 7.8, cells stop functioning and the body dies. The body therefore continually strives to balance pH. When this balance is compromised many problems can occur.

An imbalanced diet high in acidic-producing foods such as animal protein, sugar, caffeine and processed foods puts pressure on the body's regulating systems to maintain pH neutrality. The extra buffering required can deplete the body of alkaline minerals such as sodium, potassium, magnesium and calcium, making the person prone to chronic and degenerative disease. Minerals are borrowed from vital organs and bones to buffer (neutralize) the acid and safely remove it from the body. Because of this strain, the body can suffer severe and prolonged damage--a condition that may go undetected for years.

It's What You Eat, Not How Much You Eat

Weight gain can have as much to do with what you eat as how much you eat. In a recent Penn State University study, overweight people ate as many carbohydrates as they desired. As long as those carbohydrates were low glycemic index foods, they lost weight. Low glycemic index foods include whole, fresh, fiber-rich foods that are minimally processed and low in sugars and fats such as non-starchy vegetables, fresh fruits, beans and peas, 100% whole grains, nuts and dairy products.

- Low Glycemic Foods: black beans, broccoli, cherries, leafy vegetables, milk, peanuts and peanut butter, pears, plums, soybeans, tomatoes, wild rice, yogurt, whole grains.
- Moderately Low Glycemic Foods: apples, garbanzo beans (chickpeas), ice cream, navy beans, oranges, peas, pinto beans, potato chips.
- Moderately High Glycemic Index Foods: bananas, candy bars, potatoes, white pita bread, oat, oat bread, raisins, carrots, brown rice, kidney beans.

Include Exercise!

If you do not exercise, weight loss is tougher. If you live a sedentary life, your metabolism may have dropped to "starvation mode." If you reduce what you eat enough to lose weight with such low metabolism, you will not be able to get all the nutrients you need.

So while you get in the alkaline food habit, get in the exercise habit, too!

Acidosis Puts You at Risk

Acidosis can lead to many health problems in addition to weight gain. Acidosis decreases your ability to absorb nutrients, impairs cellular energy production and repair, makes your body unable to excrete certain toxins and increases your susceptibility to fatigue and illness.

Acidosis can cause:
- Cardiovascular damage.

- Diabetes.
- Gastritis, bladder and kidney problems.
- Osteoporosis, joint and muscle pain.
- Slow digestion and elimination.
- Yeast/fungal overgrowth.
- Depression and stress.
- Headaches, dental and eye problems, mouth ulcers and cracked lips.
- Unhealthy hair, skin and nails.

4

Allergies & Sweets: Sugar's Nothing to Sneeze At

A Spoonful of Sugar may help the medicine go down. But, if you eat much more than that, sugar can actually make you sick—especially if you have allergies. Sugar can provoke an inflammatory response that is identical to an allergic immune response. If you already have allergies, you may well double your misery.

Sugar suppresses your immune system. If you eat a lot of sugar, you are not only more likely to experience an allergic event, you are also less able to fight off viruses and bacterial infections.

Sugar can cause your cells to swell and aggravate allergic swelling you are already experiencing if you have an allergy.

Where Is the Sugar Hiding?

It's no surprise to read that candy, ice cream, cookies, pastries and sweet desserts have a lot of sugar. But sugar hides in a lot of other foods, as well. Did you know that a can of soda pop has about 12 teaspoons of sugar in it? Fruit juices often have a very high sugar content as well—it's usually a better idea to get your servings of fruit from a piece of fresh fruit rather than from a glass of processed juice.

Just because a product label touts it as "natural" and "healthy" does not mean it is. Read the labels! Most granola bars, flavored yogurts and yogurt smoothies, trail mixes and commercial whole grain cereals are packed with sugar.

The USDA requires manufacturers to list label ingredients in order of quantity. If the first ingredient is sugar, then there is more sugar in the product than anything else. Manufacturers think they can trick you by using many different types of sugar. That way they don't have to list any of them first. Fructose, lactose, dextrose, corn syrup, sugar, sorbitol, mannitol, malitol and xylitol are all names for sugar (the –ose suffix indicates sugar). So, the granola bar that lists whole grain as its first ingredient and follows with a list of three or four sugars may well be as sweet as cotton candy.

Sugar also hides in high-glycemic carbs like potato chips and white bread, carbs which quickly convert to sugar in your body.

Sweet Seduction

Allopathic doctors do not recognize sugar as an allergen. The rationale is that since our body breaks down our foods into glucose (blood sugar) how in the world could one be allergic to it? However, naturopathic doctors, informed nutritionists and alternative health practitioners have been warning us about the dangers of sugar for decades.

In 1954, in her landmark book, Let's Eat Right to Keep Fit, nutrition pioneer Adelle Davis wrote, "Our American diet has become largely one of sugar. To me it seems that the survival of every person unaware of nutrition is at stake . . . ."

While sugar won't cause a response on a standard allergy test, too much sugar (or high glycemic carbs) causes an inflammatory response identical to the immune response. Why? Excess sugar interferes with the absorption of vitamins and minerals crucial to healthy immune response, makes mayhem with your metabolism and disables your neurotransmitters. The energy rush and insulin spike that you get from sugar creates an imbalanced body chemistry.

Artificial Sweeteners Are Not the Answer

Many people kicking the sugar habit turn to NutraSweet (aspartame), Splenda (sucralose) or Sweet'N Low (saccharin). All of these can pose disastrous side effects. Splenda users have reported bladder pain, irritable bowel syndrome, extreme abdominal cramping, symptoms mimicking stroke and heart attack, panic attacks, painful skin rashes and life-threatening anaphylactic shock.

Saccharin causes cancer. Aspartame has a list of side effects as long as your arm, including blindness, hearing impairment, seizures, depression, irritability, hives, menstrual irregularities, hair loss and gradual weight gain.

More Sugar Dangers

If you have allergies, that's one good reason to reduce the amount of sugar in your diet. If you don't have allergies, too much sugar can still do you harm.

Other Sugar Facts:

- Sugar places major demands on your digestive system, and interferes with absorption of crucial vitamins and minerals.
- Sugar wreaks havoc on your metabolism, making it difficult for you to absorb the healthy foods you're eating.
- Sugar depletes valuable neurotransmitters that help you think clearly. Confusion, forgetfulness, ADHD, and depression are symptoms that can occur as much as 2 days after eating sugar.

- The energy rush and insulin spike that you get from sugar creates an imbalance in your body chemistry. This can lead to weight gain, insulin resistance, and loss of appetite control.
- Muscle cramping, PMS, joint pain and fatigue are other common symptoms of sugar sensitivity.

Reducing the amount of sugar you eat can be a challenge. The more you eat, the more you want! For starters, read labels so you know you aren't eating hidden sugars. Avoid sugary juices and soft drinks—opt for a glass of water with a twist of lemon. Avoid fast foods and cook from scratch when you can.

When that sugar craving raises its ugly head, try a piece of fruit or cheese. If you must give in, have a cup of herbal tea with a half-teaspoon of honey. Honey is twice as sweet as sugar and impacts blood sugar levels less dramatically. Sugar dulls your sensitivity to the natural sugars in fruit. After you kick your sugar habit, fruit may taste better than ever. The more fruit you eat, the better!

Building resistance to allergies is all about building better overall health. Your health is what you eat. Note: organic foods do not contain the preservatives and colorings that aggravate your hay fever, allergic rhinitis and other allergies.

Here are a few helpful guidelines:

1. Select organic fruit and vegetables whenever possible. Wash or peel non-organic produce.
2. Choose fruits and vegetables in season. This limits your exposure to the chemicals used to delay ripening, prolong shelf-life, preserve color and so on.
3. Eat whole grains. They carry a lower glycemic load (convert to sugar slower) and give you more vitamins, minerals and protein.
4. Supplement your diet with antioxidant nutrients: vitamins

A, C, and E, and the minerals zinc and selenium. Since the detoxification of many pesticides involves these nutrients.

5. Eliminate milk and other dairy products, especially if they are not organic. Know your producer! The USDA allows some so-called organic factory farms to raise dairy cattle on pesticide contaminated feed, hormones and antibiotics as long as the animals are on an organic diet when they begin giving milk.

5

Alzheimer's Disease: Strategies to Remember

Every hour, 330 American baby boomers turn 60. Every 72 seconds, another one of them develops Alzheimer's disease. More than 5 million American seniors currently suffer with Alzheimer's. Experts project that the number will rise to 16 million by 2050. What is causing this epidemic of dementia?

Many experts agree that the American lifestyle and diet are contributing factors to Alzheimer's. So, too, are certain prescription medications. For example, the drug Detrol, prescribed for overactive bladder and incontinence, causes dementia that is often misdiagnosed as Alzheimer's disease. (The "disease" overactive bladder is really no disease at all. The condition was invented by Detrol's manufacturer to boost sales!)

In addition, prescription drugs used to treat Alzheimer's Disease provide little help or hope. The blockbuster drug, Aricept, brings its makers nearly $2 billion a year in sales but does little for the Alzheimer's patients taking it ($1,500 a year for each individual patient taking it). Aricept's common side effects include vomiting, dizziness and insomnia. Physicians often prescribe antidepressants, tranquilizers and anti-psychotic medications to patients with Alzheimer's. These too do very little to ameliorate the condition but do indeed expose the patient to a wide range of potentially dangerous side effects.

Avoiding Alzheimer's

Ensuring good overall health is also the best way to avoid Alzheimer's. Eat wholesome, God-made foods: fruits, vegetables, whole grains and healthy fats, like almonds, walnuts and the fish oils found in salmon and other cold water fish. People who eat fish one time a week reduce risks of Alzheimer's by 50%. Half of your brain is fat. Eating bad fats can hurt your brain while eating good fats can help it. Go easy on red meat and egg yolks.

Phase out fast foods and prepared foods that offer you a long list of chemical ingredients. Drinking plenty of water every day also helps brain function. Did you know that most children's bodies are 75% water while most elderly folks are only 50%? Stay hydrated and age more slowly.

Exercise your brain and your body! Physical exercise helps balance your blood sugar. High blood sugar and insulin levels, as well as diabetes, are associated with increased risk of Alzheimer's disease. It's never too late to start exercising. Try walking or, if you have arthritis, water aerobics. Tai chi is another excellent exercise for older adults.

Brain Exercises

- For starters, one of the best ways you can exercise your brain is to turn off the TV and engage in the real world. In addition:
- Read
- Do brain games like crossword puzzles, sodoku or picture puzzles.
- Play chess, cards, dominoes or other board games that require mental focus

Supplementation

Ask your alternative healthcare provider for proper dosages of the following supplements which have been proven to help prevent Alzheimer's disease:

- Fish oil capsules
- Vitamin E
- Vitamin C
- B vitamins, especially folic acid
- Beta-carotene
- NAC (N-acetyl-cysteine)
- ALA (Alpha lipoic acid)
- ALC (Acetyl-L-carnitine)
- CoQ10 (Coenzyme Q10)

In addition, use curry and turmeric spices to flavor your favorite home-cooked dishes. Both have proven brain health benefits.

In conclusion

If you or someone you love has been diagnosed with Alzheimer's disease, take these positive steps:

- Build brain power, through exercise, good nutrition and supplementation.
- Investigate prescription medications. Their side effects might be the real culprit in dementia.

Find support. Alzheimer's devastates relationships and gobbles up financial resources. Find friends at church or a support group through your local Alzheimer's organization to help you cope. As doctors suggest expensive drug therapies, be aware that these will not cure Alzheimer's and may not even help slow its progression. If the medication isn't working, don't be afraid to terminate its use.

6

Asthma: Foods that Soothe, Foods to Avoid

Do you have asthma? Does your child have asthma? Then you have experienced the terror and irritation that happens when airways become so sensitive and swollen that you cough, wheeze and can't catch your breath. Asthma symptoms can be triggered by exercise, cold air, toxins such as allergens, pollutants, viruses, and food.

Detoxify Your World

We live in a toxic world. The air we breathe contains pollutants and viruses. The water we drink may have chlorine, fluoride and other decontaminants added. Our bodies work hard to eliminate these toxins from our systems. But sometimes, there are just too many. You reach the point where that last toxic straw breaks your immune system's back. If you're like 20 million other Americans, your body reacts with an asthma attack.

The first step to having fewer asthma attacks is to avoid toxins. I realize this may be easier said than done. However, do your best to avoid situations and environments where you'll run into the allergens that trigger your attacks. During pollen seasons or on ozone action days, stay indoors or wear a protective mask.

In your home, try to keep allergens, dust and dust mites at bay.

- Use air filtration and houseplants to cleanse indoor air. Don't forget to throw the windows open now and then to freshen the air, as well.
- Wash your bedding in hot water every week.
- Brush your pets daily to reduce the amount of dander floating about.
- Use non-toxic, "Green" cleaning products—or good old baking soda and vinegar—in your home. Avoid

commercial air fresheners.

- Paint your walls with low VOC ratings and avoid those plastics and furnishings which emit chemical gases.

The next step is to detoxify your body

For starters, drink 8 to 12 glasses of PURE water every day. Your best water source may well be your own tap as long as you have attached a filtration system that specifically filters out fluoride and other contaminants. Plastic water bottles not only overburden our landfills, they also emit small amounts of toxins into the water they hold.

Colon cleansing can also help detoxify your body. An easy and practical way to keep your colon clean is to eat more high fiber foods (whole grains, fresh fruits and raw vegetables) while avoiding processed foods and sugar.

Better BrEAThing: What You Eat and Asthma Control

Did you know food allergies are a major trigger for asthma attacks? The standard American diet of refined, packaged, additive-ridden processed foods aggravates asthma. These foods lack the nutrients you need to build your health—and contain

The following chart details common food additives that aggravate asthma.

Calcium benzoate	In drinks, low-sugar products, cereals, meats.	Aggravates hay fever, hives and asthma.
Calcium sulphite	Many foods.	Aggravates bronchial problems, asthma and cardiovascular problems.

....

Sodium metabisulphite	Many foods.	Provokes life-threatening asthma.
Sulphur dioxide	Many foods.	Causes bronchial problems in those with asthma or low blood pressure.
Brilliant Black BN Allura RedAC Ponceau 4R, Conchineal, Red A Sunset Yellow FCF, Orange Yellow S Tartrazine	Many foods.	Aggravates asthma symptoms.

In a clinical study of children with life-threatening asthma, more than 50% were found to have food allergies, especially to peanuts, compared to only 10% in the control group. This posed the possibility that life-threatening asthma attacks are triggered by food allergies.

Other foods that commonly cause food allergies are: cow's milk, wheat, yeast, eggs, sugar, soy, corn and chocolate. Pulse testing or an elimination diet can help you determine which foods cause you or your child to have an asthma attack.

Foods that Relieve and Prevent Asthma

When your body is well nourished, your immune system has the natural power it needs to handle toxins and allergens. These foods have been proven to help your immune system relieve and prevent asthma attacks:

- Fresh, organic fruits and vegetables in generous amounts.
- 100% whole grains: breads, cereal, pasta and crackers.
- Cold water fish: cod, salmon, mackerel, halibut, salmon, tuna, sardines and herring.
- Extra virgin olive oil
- Flax seeds or flax seed oil
- Herbal spices: rosemary, ginger and turmeric

Picture a mixed greens salad with olive oil and balsamic vinegar accompanying a juicy, pink salmon steak baked with fresh rosemary and served on a plate of tender steamed vegetables and some sweet, ripe fruit. A satisfying meal like this is ideal if you have asthma.

Why Organic?

Eating organic foods will help you avoid the food additives that trigger asthma as well as pesticide residues which also trigger asthma attacks. In fact, eating organic can be a matter of life and breath for asthma sufferers.

Approximately 89% to 99% of all fresh fruits, grains and vegetables are sprayed with pesticides. In random testing, some fruits—particularly strawberries, raspberries, grapes and tomatoes—had residues of at least six different pesticides! Carrots and lettuce were found to have pesticide residue levels up to 25 times higher than the USDA safety limit. Pesticides are used to treat animal feed, contaminating most meat, milk and dairy products.

1. Select organic fruit and vegetables whenever possible. Wash or peel non-organic produce.
2. Choose fruits and vegetables in season. This means that your exposure to the chemicals used to delay ripening, prolong shelf-life, preserve color and so on, will be limited.

4. Eliminate milk and other dairy products, especially if they are not organic. Know your producer! The USDA allows some so-called organic factory farms to raise dairy cattle on pesticide contaminated feed, hormones and antibiotics as long as the animals are on an organic diet when they begin giving milk.

Did you know that people who embark on a vegetarian diet usually relieve their allergy symptoms within 12 months?

Help Your Foods Help Your Body

Because of the ways our foods are processed and delivered, they often lose the essential phytonutrients we need to maintain health. That's why it's important to supplement your diet with quality grade nutraceutical products that are targeted to your individual health needs. If you or someone you love has asthma, consider supplementation.

- As a preventive measure, take a good, natural (not synthetic) multi-vitamin that provides generous quantities of vitamin A, B6, B12, C, and E; the minerals zinc, magnesium and selenium; and antioxidants and bioflavanoids.
- Aloe vera and garlic can help balance and fortify the immune system.
- Flax or fish oil can reduce the inflammatory-allergic response.

7
Bladder Infection: Common Sense Care

Affecting more women than men, bladder infections cause pain, discomfort, inconvenience and, if left untreated, a more serious infection that can migrate into the kidneys. Bladder infections are common among women today for a variety of reasons.

What You Eat and Drink

If evil scientists were looking for a way to cause an epidemic of bladder infections in a population, they would have to look no further than the standard American diet. Sugar, refined carbohydrates (which convert to sugar in the body) and the hosts of chemical additives all set the bladder up for infection. Both regular and diet soda pop promote bladder infection.

Plus, when it comes to soda pop, you introduce two more badder-bladder factors: caffeine and sodium benzoate. Both act as diuretics, drying up your poor bladder so it has no choice but to strike back.

If you want to quit having those constant bladder infections, kick the sugar habit. drink pure water instead of soda pop, sugary juices or artificially sweetened beverages and change up to 100% whole grain breads and pastas.

What You Don't Drink

Most of us don't drink enough water—for adults, that is eight to twelve 8-ounce glasses a day.

What You Wear

Another enemy of the woman's bladder is constrictive clothing made of synthetic fabric. Tight, polyester pants and nylon panty hose restrict air flow and encourage bacteria to grow. These bacteria can back up into the bladder through the urethra. Thong underwear also encourages this kind of contamination.

Wear looser pants or skirts, cotton underwear and avoid panty hose, if possible.

Hygiene

From the time they are toddlers, girls should be taught to wipe their bottoms from front to back after bowel movements. Bacteria from the bowel movements can be introduced into the bladder via the urethral opening when girls wipe back to front.

Bubble bath has also been implicated as a cause of bladder infections, especially among little girls.

If you have a bladder infection now, these tips may help clear it up more quickly:

- Empty your bladder often . . . don't "hold it."
- Empty your bladder before and after intercourse.
- Drink a glass of water every waking hour
- Eat fresh parsley and celery to increase urine flow.
- Cranberry juice makes bladder walls slippery (a good thing). However, try to find unsweetened cranberry juice or herbal cranberry tea as sugar and artificial sweeteners can worsen your condition.
- Avoid all sugar, alcohol, carbonated drinks, chocolate, caffeine and processed foods.
- Alkalize your urine by taking ½ tsp. of baking soda in a glass of water twice a day.
- Add a good source of L. acidophilus to your diet.
- The herb Uva Ursi acts as a natural diuretic to get infection out. Aloe vera juice (1 to 3 ounces daily) and Echinacea can boost immune system response.
- Supplement with a high quality multivitamin and mineral formula daily.

Cancer and Self Care

If you or a loved one have been diagnosed with cancer, you may feel like life is spinning totally out of control. You are probably shuffling to countless doctors' appointments, undergoing a host of unfamiliar procedures and ingesting medications with names that are hard to pronounce. You may feel like a stranger in a strange land. You are even learning a new language. While the temptation may be to give up and give yourself over to your medical team, remember, no one cares about your condition more than you do. By taking responsibility for your own healthcare, researching alternatives and taking some basic steps in self care, you will increase your chances of beating cancer and getting your life back.

Basic Lifestyle Guidelines

If you were eating a good, healthy, natural, organic diet before your diagnosis of cancer, now is no time to abandon it. If you were not, now is the time to start. Many cancer patients have found that switching up their nutrition has made a huge difference in their outcome and Quality of Life.

- Eat whole, raw foods as often as possible: organically grown fruits, vegetables and whole grains.
- Drink 8 glasses of pure filtered water every day.
- Include a tablespoon of flaxseed oil daily for essential fatty acids (EFAs).
- Take a natural vitamin-mineral supplement.

In addition, it will be helpful if you observe a three- to five-day juice fast once every six months. For three days, drink only freshly juiced organic vegetables and fruits along with plenty of pure, filtered water.

Say "Absolutely No" to:
- Fried foods.
- Meat and dairy products.
- Alcohol and smoking.
- Artificial food colorings or flavorings and preservatives.
- Processed foods are strictly forbidden. Eat nothing that says enriched, fortified, bleached *etc.* on the label.

Detoxify

Detoxification is a natural function addressed by many of your body systems. However, sometimes the toxic overload is too much for the body to handle. Both the causes and medical cures of your cancer may build up toxins in your body. Routine detoxification supports your body in its fight to rid you of substances and by-products that impair your health, specifically the immune system.

For starters, clean and replenish your G.I. tract. More than one half of the immune system operates from here.

- Use an herbal-fiber bowel restorer to encourage at least two bowel movements daily (for normal colon function).
- Supplement with digestive enzymes and probiotics, *e.g.* acidophilus.
- Lose excess fat; that's where toxins hide.
- Support liver and kidney function with the herb, milk thistle, and greens.

Fortify

Cancer and its treatments really pack a wallop when it comes to your immune system. You do not have to sit back and let your immune system deteriorate. You can take steps to strengthen it.

- Learn to relax. Stress is the immune system's #1 enemy. Walk every day, if you can. Connect with nature. Schedule a regular therapeutic massage.
- Get plenty of rest, exercise, sunshine and fresh air.
- Eat properly: fruits vegetables, whole grains, water.
- Exercise consistently to move immune fluid (general recommendation: 30 minutes, 3-5 five times a week). Brisk walking is great!
- Increase antioxidant levels with 4 glasses of green tea or juice with green powder, wheat grass, or barley grass daily.

If you are undergoing chemotherapy:

- Take balanced multiple vitamin/mineral supplement. This is of the utmost importance!
- Avoid meat and dairy. Concentrate on raw fruits and vegetables (juicing is best), whole grains and natural non-processed foods. Dietary changes are a must!
- Get plenty of rest. Aloe juice every day will help rebuild the immune system. Get plenty of fluids, especially pure filtered water.
- Eat 10 raw almonds a day. They contain an important ingredient that is toxic to cancer cells but not to normal cells. This also applies to other nuts and seeds—especially apricot seeds!

Science and Supplementation

Some physicians still operate under the false notion that supplements can interfere with chemotherapy. This misconception was dispelled in the early 1990s by oncologist Charles Simone, M.D. in his landmark book, *Cancer and Nutrition*. Citing numerous references, he states, "All studies show that vitamins and minerals do not interfere with the anti-tumor effects of chemotherapy or radiation therapy. In fact, on the contrary, some vitamins and minerals used in conjunction with chemotherapy and/or radiation therapy have been shown to protect normal tissue and potentiate

Physicians have taken an anti-supplement stance in the past because of an overall bias against supplements as well as a misguided belief that chemotherapy kills cancer by inflicting oxidative, free-radical damage. However, University of Kansas School of Medicine professor and researcher, Jeanne Drisko, M.D., has shown that chemotherapy actually causes cancer cells, in layman's terms, "to commit suicide."

In fact, while supplement use during chemotherapy has no downside, it does have tremendous benefits. Chemotherapy compromises the immune system and often is associated with extreme malnutrition. Supplements address both of these potentially dangerous side effects.

Christ Is the "Cancer Answer."

Yes, even cancer cells can be overcome! You simply need to equip your immune system with the tools it needs to wage war against cancer and other diseases—and win. Terrible fear grips most people when they hear the word *cancer*, but cancer is not the "Big C" word, Christ Jesus is! He's the "Cancer Answer."

If you've already been diagnosed with cancer or another life-threatening or debilitating illness, your body may have lost a battle, but that doesn't mean you've lost the war! You can begin turning the tide of battle today. Start with believing God's Word when it says "by His stripes we are healed" (Isaiah 53:5). Search Scripture for other passages that promise healing and wholeness for the children of God—there are many—and begin speaking them over your life daily. Then take a closer look at how God designed your immune system.

Did you know the average person's body experiences two thousand cancerous changes *daily*? A cancer cell is one that starts dividing uncontrollably, and that happens two thousand times a day in everyone. Did you know most people actually develop about half a dozen tumors in their lifetimes that doctors could detect if they examined the right place at the right time? Yet not everyone gets diagnosed with cancer every day or undergoes cancer treatment six times in their lives. Why not? Because the immune system is specifically designed to stop the spread of cancer and other diseases.

Sickness is no match for strong immune systems in detoxified bodies!

"T4 Killer Cells," the white blood cells in the immune system, rid people's bodies of cancerous cells and malicious invaders like viruses and bacteria. T4 cells resemble Pac-Man in the old game where Pac-Man goes around gobbling up everything in his path.

That's a picture of God's chemotherapy and radiation treatment happening daily in each of us.

If your body hasn't stayed on top of cancerous changes or hasn't successfully warded off other illnesses, it's time to confess the Word of God for healing and give your body some new tools to use in waging war on disease.

9

Chronic Fatigue and Fibromyalgia: Syndromes with Solutions

More than 800,000 people in the U.S. suffer with the debilitating symptoms of CFS. Another 5 million have been diagnosed with FMS.

If you have CFS or FMS, you may experience:
- Loss of healthful, deep sleep patterns.
- Hormone imbalances.
- Lingering flu symptoms.
- Irritable bowel syndrome.
- Headaches, facial and body pain.
- Heightened sensitivity to light, noise, touch and odors.
- Exhaustion.
- Swelling and tenderness in your lymph glands.

Do Chronic Fatigue and Fibromyalgia Syndromes Share a Common Cause?

Many experts contend that Chronic Fatigue Syndrome (CFS) and Fibromyalgia Syndrome (FMS) share more than some common symptoms. These conditions may also share a common cause—and in fact be a progression of the same disorder.

Dr. Derek Enlander, a physician treating CFS and FMS patients in New York City and faculty member at Mt. Sinai Medical Center, believes that CFS and FMS are related illnesses. "Whatever initiates the beginning of the illness then directly affects the immune system into an up-regulated or a deregulated condition," he stated. "The body, trying to heal itself and return to a natural balance, seems to constantly be adjusting to find that balance."

In years past, CFS and FMS were thought to be imaginary illnesses; their symptoms seemed to have no logical explanation and most patients experiencing the conditions were women. Though now recognized by the medical community, hard facts as to their cause and treatment are still few and far between. However, recent research has uncovered some amazing discoveries.

Mike O' Who? Mycoplasma

A specific mycoplasma was discovered to be one common cause of CFS and FMS in research by Dr. Garth Nicolson, Chief Scientific Officer and Research Professor with The Institute for Molecular Medicine and his co-researchers, Dr. Nancy L. Nicolson and Dr. Darryl See.

Mycoplasmas are the smallest self-replicating organisms known to science. Hundreds of types of mycoplasmas can be found in plants, insects and animals, but only a few are found in the human body. Not all mycoplasmas cause disease. But some do. For example, M. pneumoniae causes walking pneumonia.

Dr. Garth Nicolson explains, "Once in the cell, they steal lipids (fats) like cholesterol from the mitochondria, the components of a cell that produces energy. This makes the mitochondria 'leaky,' and they lose electrons. This is similar to a battery running down when the insulation around the battery is removed. This may be why patients with intracellular pathogenic mycoplasmas are almost always fatigued. They have run their cellular batteries down, so that less high energy molecules are available, and they are exhausted at the cellular level."

These researchers agree that long-term anti-microbials should be initiated to treat mycoplasmal infections. They also recommend boosting the immune system and supplementing with essential nutrients and vitamins.

"We always try to use the least toxic approaches in working with pathologies, so we use a lot of natural products," Dr. See said. Examples include probiotics and undenatured whey protein isolates for supporting the GI tract. This combination helps prevent overgrowth of undesirable microorganisms.

CFS and FMS may share other common causes, as well.

Those with these conditions often have lower than normal serotonin levels, hence, they have problems sleeping. Hypothyroidism (underactive thyroid) may also play a role. Chronic yeast overgrowth (Candida albicans) has also been cited as a culprit. Since CFS and FMS sufferers are more prone to infections, they may be prescribed antibiotics frequently. Antibiotics stimulate yeast overgrowth and a vicious cycle begins.

Treating any of these causes individually may help relieve your symptoms. Select herbs and foods that will help bring your body back into balance. Raw whole foods are best, especially vegetables.

Good nutrition is also a must. Fast foods and processed foods are stripped of their original nutrients—nutrients vital to health.

Drug Dangers

If you suffer with CFS or FMS, chances are your doctor has prescribed medications to help you deal with your symptoms. Be aware that both over-the-counter and prescription medications may cause you to experience potentially dangerous and painful side effects.

- Aspirin, Ibuprofen (Motrin, Advil, Nuprin, Rufin)

and Naproxen (Aleve, Naprosyn, Naprelan, Anaprox) may trigger gastrointestinal problems, ulcers, internal bleeding, increased blood pressure, dizziness, tinnitus, headaches, rashes and depression.

- Celebrex, Vioxx and Bextra can increase risk of heart attack, adversely affect digestion and kidney function and increase blood pressure. Anti-inflammatories such as Meloxicam (Mobic) may increase risk of heart attack, adversely affect kidney function and increase blood pressure.
- Tricyclic antidepressants can cause dry mouth, restlessness, reduced sexual drive, increased heart rate, constipation and possible death by overdose. And cortisol, steroidal hormone supplements and hydrocortisone can cause insomnia, weight gain and suppressed adrenal gland function.

10
Cholesterol: Finding Balance

Cholesterol is not the enemy. In fact, it is an essential, water-insoluble body nutrient closely related to vitamin D. The healthy human body produces 2,000 milligrams of cholesterol a day. When you eat foods with more cholesterol, your body slows production. When you eat less, your body compensates by producing more. It is transported inside lipoproteins, two that are prominently referred to are: low density lipoproteins (LDL) and high-density lipoproteins (HDL). Cholesterol transported from the liver by LDL regenerates new cell membranes. Old cholesterol is transported to the liver by HDL to be recycled.

Cholesterol actually plays many roles in good health:
- It holds cell walls together.
- Several hormones, including testosterone and estrogen,

are derived from cholesterol.
- Brain cells are made of cholesterol.
- It enables brain synapses to form and fire.
- Psychomotor skills depend on cholesterol.
- It patches damage to arterial walls caused by acid pH.
- It enables cell signaling for guiding and growing nerve axons.
- Cholesterol saves lives!

Is there such a thing as high cholesterol?

Yes, there is. As with sugar or calories, you can overindulge. A diet too rich in cholesterol may well raise your serum cholesterol level. However, statin drugs do not always succeed in lowering cholesterol. And when they do, those levels can be brought down too low, resulting in:
- Ischemic strokes (80% of all strokes are ischemic; 20% are hemorrhagic and linked to high cholesterol).
- Behavioral problems and depression due to lowered serotonin, a neurotransmitter in the brain.
- Learning disabilities among children.

In fact, studies reveal that elderly patients with both low cholesterol and albumin (a blood protein) are 3.5 times more likely to die before than those with normal levels.

As organizations like the National Cholesterol Education Program, the American Heart Association, National Heart, Lung and Blood Institute and American College of Cardiology set ever lower acceptable cholesterol levels, these facts are being ignored. Instead, recommendations are being made that anyone with high or moderate *risk* of developing high cholesterol be prescribed statins—Lipitor, Crestor, Lescol, Mevacor and Zocor, to name a few. Some are even being prescribed for children. While some health practitioners warn statins should not be prescribed at all, the mainstream still buckles under the influence of the pharmaceutical companies' dollars.

Achieving balance

- Cholesterol is necessary in the right amounts and in proper balance (HDL to LDL). To achieve balance, you must:
- Feed your body the nutrients it needs to balance itself. For starters, look to the foods you eat. Try to build your diet around whole, organic foods, eaten raw or cooked from scratch. Recent studies confirm that a fiber-rich diet reduces the occurrence of clogged arteries, heart disease and high cholesterol. General guidelines recommend 20 to 35 grams of fiber per day in the form of fruits, vegetables, beans and whole grains.
- Get fit. A regular fitness routine can help balance cholesterol levels.

Avoid fluoride. Your cholesterol level may also be tied to the water you drink and the toothpaste you use. A new National Research Council report on fluoride shows that fluoride, consumed at the levels in fluoridated water, can elevate blood cholesterol levels excessively.

11

Ear Infections: Common Sense Care

Ear infections are very common among children these days. Many of these infections can be linked to the child's diet. Food allergies, especially to milk and dairy products, are major causes often overlooked by pediatricians and family doctors. If your child has ear infections often, try eliminating dairy from his diet completely and see what happens. If the ear infections persist, use an elimination diet or pulse testing to see if other foods may be at the root of the problem.

Ear infections, as well as cold, flu and other illnesses, can also be the result of poor nutrition or too much sugar in the diet. Sugar compromises the immune system. Did you ever notice that a lot of children get sick after Halloween or the Christmas holidays—after celebrations that include even more sugar than they eat during other times of the year? Get your family out of the sugar habit and watch their health improve!

Here are some more helpful tips for preventing and treating ear infection:

- Schedule a spinal adjustment to ensure cervical alignment.
- Avoid cow's milk, wheat, yeast, eggs, corn, sugar, oranges and peanut butter, if allergies are suspected..
- Use colloidal silver and garlic to fight infection naturally.
- Build the immune system with a raw fruit, vegetable and whole grain diet.
- Supplement with a high quality multi-vitamin/mineral and aloe vera.
- Increase good bacteria in the body by supplementing with L. acidophilus (especially important if antibiotics have been used.)
- Feed infants with ear infections in an upright position to help eustachian tubes to drain.
- Avoid cigarette smoke.
- Insert a few drops of warm garlic or olive oil in the ear canal. Or use a commercial herbal ear oil with willow bark, olive oil and garlic.
- Avoid antibiotics, antihistamines and decongestants. These drugs suppress normal immune response and lead to relapse.
- Increase fluids, especially water. Children should drink at least 8 glasses of water a day even when they are not ill.
- Drink 1 –2 ounces of aloe vera juice with immune stimulating herbs each day.

12

Endometriosis: End It Once and for All

A painful condition, endometriosis is caused by an abnormal growth of tissue outside of the uterus. If you live with endometriosis, these tips may help.

Nutrition

Upgrade to a whole foods diet that is based on fresh fruits, vegetables and whole grains. Avoid meat and dairy products, especially those from animals treated with antibiotics or fed hormones.

Supplement your diet with an all natural, balanced multivitamin/mineral formula that contains absorbable sources of calcium and magnesium.

Include flax seed oil in your diet every day. You can use it on salads or stirred into oatmeal or take one to three 1,000 mg capsules daily.

Other helpful supplements include: aloe vera juice, garlic, astralagus, pau d'arco, red clover, and alfalfa, for Vitamin K and iron.

Detoxification

Detoxifying your body is especially important for women with endometriosis. For starters, drink at least ten glasses of pure filtered water every day. Include many high fiber foods in your diet to keep toxins moving through and out of your body.

Fasting for three days each month before the beginning of your period is beneficial. Fast on steamed distilled water and freshly juiced fruit and vegetable juices.

Avoid toxins in your environment, especially dioxins (which can leech from plastic water bottles and dinnerware when frozen or micro-waved), dry cleaning fluids, pesticides and drugs. The chlorine bleaching process used to whiten paper, rayon cotton and materials most tampons are made of also can contaminate you with dioxins.

Exercise

Consistent exercise, best started when you are in your early 20s, can decrease estrogen and lessen incidence of endometriosis. However, it's never too late to start a sensible exercise program.

Remedies

Natural progesterone cream used from ovulation till the first day of your period can help balance estrogen levels.

13

Flu and Common Cold: Common Sense Care

Caused by more than 200 different viruses that attack the upper respiratory tract, the common cold can cause sneezing, watery eyes, runny nose, coughing and other irritating symptoms. Healthy adults usually fight these viruses at least once or twice a year if their immune systems are weak.

When you get a cold and fight it off, this shows your immune system is working. If it takes more than a day or two, your immune system may be compromised.

Because children's immune systems are still maturing, they may fight colds off a little more often than adults.

Shorten and Win the Fight!

- **Remain active without overdoing it.** The immune system has no pump. Activity moves immune fluids through your body. Walking or light exercise actually

helps fight off a cold!
- **Double your daily dose of multiple vitamins and minerals.** Make sure your multi has adequate vitamin C and zinc.
- **Take Echinacea at the first sign of symptoms** (echinacea augustfolia is the preferred extract for colds and flu.)
- **Increase fluids**, especially pure water with lemon. Sip hot liquids; potato peeling broth is great.
- **Wash your hands** often so you don't spread the virus.
- **Avoid over-the-counter remedies**, which block normal body functions and hinder immune system activity.
- **Do not take antibiotics.** They are only effective on specific bacteria, not on viruses that cause cold and flu. Use colloidal silver, garlic and cayenne pepper as natural alternatives.

Influenza

A highly contagious viral infection spread by coughing and sneezing, the "flu" infects the upper respiratory tract. When you come down with the flu, you usually experience a dry throat, cough and body aches. You do not feel like doing much of anything, even eating. The flu is more serious in folks who are 65 or older.

When you have the flu, you can follow the previously listed recommendations for care of the common cold with one exception—do not remain active. In addition:
- Get plenty of rest.
- Boost your immune system with fresh fruit and vegetable juices.
- Brew and drink peppermint tea to open nasal passages.
- Use cayenne pepper to keep mucous flowing (mucous flow helps eliminate the virus.)
- Do not try to lower a fever under 102°. Increased body temperature helps inactivate the virus and speeds up

immune system function.
- For sore throat, gargle. Alternate warm water with hot salt water several times a day. (1/4 tsp. salt per 8 oz. water)
- Cough! Cover your mouth and let it happen. This is your body's way of expelling the virus.

Homemade Healthy Cough Syrup

If your cough interferes with sleep, use this homemade cough syrup as an alternative to the toxic OTC remedies sold by the pharmacy.

1/2 tsp. slippery elm bark powder
1/4 C. honey
1/2 C. boiling water

Add slippery elm powder and honey to boiling water. Stir well. Take 1 tsp. every 3 hours.

14
Gout and the Foods that Soothe It

What is gout?

Gout, hyperuricemia, is a painful inflammation caused by uric acid build-up in the joints. It occurs when the liver produces more uric acid than the kidneys can excrete in the urine. Over time, the uric acid crystallizes and settles in the joints—most often the big toe or ankle--causing swelling, inflammation, stiffness and pain. Over time, the uric acid crystals can damage your nerves, cartilage and bone.

Gout can be caused by eating too many rich foods or drinking alcohol. Gout is also a side effect of prescription drugs used to treat high blood pressure, high cholesterol and digestive upsets. No wonder more than two million people in the U.S. suffer with gout.

If you have gout, you've probably been told to avoid certain rich foods and alcohol. Did you know there are also foods that help relieve gout symptoms?

Life is a Bowl of Cherries.

Researchers have found that eating six to eight fresh cherries a day, in between meals, alleviates gout symptoms. If you feel a gout attack coming on, eat 20 to 30 cherries immediately.

Cherries help support the health of the connective tissue that is damaged by gout; they have an enzyme that neutralizes uric acid; and they help prevent inflammation. Frozen and canned cherries can be used but watch the sugar and additive content. A cup of strawberries, a cup of blueberries or a tablespoon of black cherry juice concentrate with each meal may help, as well.

In fact, eating generous amounts of any fresh **fruits and vegetables** can keep uric acid crystals from depositing in the joints. Grapes help your body to eliminate uric acid from your body before it has a chance to crystallize. The potassium in other high fiber foods can do the same: baked potatoes with skin, yams, spinach, dried peaches or prunes, avocados,cantaloupes, kidney or lima beans, bananas, orange juice and carrots.

Drink to Your Health

While you may have been cautioned to quit toasting with alcohol, you can make your gout better with the following beverages. Make them a ritual—serve in a cocktail glass, on the rocks or with a twist.

Water. All of us need to drink six to eight, eight-ounce glasses of water every day. If you have gout, drinking enough water is even more important. You may also want to include fresh fruit juices and herbal teas rather than soda pop or caffeinated beverages that drive water and minerals from your body. Keeping your urine diluted helps you to excrete uric acid before crystals have a chance to form.

Lemon juice can prevent gout attacks. Drink the juice of one freshly squeezed lemon in a glass of lukewarm water after every meal. It helps your body neutralize acid, the uric acid that triggers gout attacks. (To get more juice out from the lemon, bring it to room temperature and roll it on the counter before juicing.).

Celery seed tea. As another gout preventative, cook a tablespoon of celery seeds in two cups of water till soft; strain and drink 1/2 cup four times a day.

Apple cider vinegar and raw honey. Mix two teaspoons of each in a glass of water and drink at mealtime.

A word of caution to dieters

Severe dieting or fasting can create excess lactic acid. Lactic acid impairs the kidneys so that they cannot excrete uric acid— ouch! More gout pain! Crash diets can also drive potassium from your body and increase uric acid formation. If you need to lose weight, follow a sensible diet that includes smaller portions of a variety of healthy, whole foods.

Herbal "Wonder Food" Remedies

The FDA has issued warnings about many common over the counter and prescription pain relievers. As Parts 1 and 2 showed you, certain foods can help prevent and relieve your gout pain. So can some herbal remedies and vitamin/mineral supplements. The following have been commonly used by people with gout.

Take these herbs as a tea or extract as directed:

- Alfalfa

- Bilberry

- Black cohosh

- Buchu tea

- Devil's claw

- Garlic

- Hawthorn

- Hydrangea

- Nettle

- Parsley

- Red clover

- Saffron

- Yarrow with Nettle

Use these herbs in a poultice:

- Castor oil. Warm and soak into a piece of flannel and apply to affected area, one hour twice daily.
- Cayenne pepper. Boil one tablespoon in 1 cup of vinegar and 1 cup of water. Dab onto painful joint. Or mix with wintergreen oil to make a paste and apply.
- Charcoal. One cup with 3 tablespoons of ground flaxseed and warm water.
- Ginger. Mix 1/3 cup ground ginger your bath; soak 30 minutes. Rinse well to avoid skin irritation.

- Mullein. Soak leaves in a hot vinegar/water mixture. Pack on the affected area.
- Spearmint. Using leaves, wrap affected area.
- Rose hips. Boil in apple cider vinegar and dab on affected area.

Take these supplements as directed:

- B complex

- Bromelain

- Fish oil capsules

- L-glutamine

- L-glutathione

- L-glycine

- L-methionine

- Magnesium citrate

- Quercetin

- Shark cartilage

- Vitamin C

- Vitamin E

Build good health with good nutrition.

Like all health issues, gout will improve as your overall health improves. So, maintain a healthy weight and exercise daily. Eat healthy foods. A diet that includes plenty of fresh fruits, vegetables and whole grains helps control uric acid levels.

If possible, consume natural, organic foods, raw or prepared from scratch. And, as your healthcare provider has probably told you, avoid those foods known to instigate gout flare-ups: scallops, shrimp, sardines, red meat, gravy, cream sauces, sweets, ice cream, organ meats, turkey, dried peas, legumes, fried foods, caffeine and alcohol.

Pressure Points

Are you still experiencing gout pain? Apply some pressure:

- Press just below the center of your nose toward the upper lip.
- Massage between the ball of your foot and the bottom of your big toe on each foot. On the left foot only, stimulate a point halfway between the base of the little toe and the heel pad.
- Press inward and upward at the base of the skull.

15
Heartburn and Acid Reflux Help

If you suffer with heartburn, acid reflux, diarrhea, constipation, gas, irritable bowel syndrome (IBS) or other digestive upsets, you may be spending a lot of money on over-the-counter and prescription remedies to treat your painful symptoms. The trouble is, symptoms are only a signal—a way your body communicates that something is not right. Taking a Tums or popping a Zelnorm may make you feel better temporarily, but such measures do not address the root cause. In fact, masking symptoms—and ignoring what your body is trying to tell you—can cause health problems to escalate.

Fooling Your Body Never Fixes Anything

Your digestive system takes charge of a miraculously interactive process that releases and absorbs nutrients from the foods you eat, nutrients needed for healthy living.

In the mouth, enzymes in saliva begin breaking down food. In the stomach, acid and enzymes break down foods, releasing vitamins, minerals, protein and fats. Pancreatic juices and bile from the gall bladder get in on the act, too. A phenomenal relationship between the brain and the gut takes place on a molecular level as neuropeptides and serotonins guide absorption of the released nutrients traveling through the intestines.

Without well-absorbed nutrients, none of the body's systems can enjoy optimum health. When the digestive system is out of balance, it belches, burns, cramps, holds in or explodes.

It's important to listen to what the body is trying to tell you—not shut it up with prescription drugs or over-the-counter remedies.

Acid Reflux

Acid reflux disease (Reflux Esophagitis) is a digestive disorder of epidemic proportions. One out of ten Americans suffer from its symptoms. One drug used to treat it, Prilosec, is the top selling drug in the world.

Heartburn and acid reflux occur when gastric (stomach) juices back up into the esophagus. Overeating or eating foods which relax the lower muscles of the esophagus can cause reflux. Other causes include a diet high in junk, fast and processed foods and use of medications.

Most remedies for acid reflux and heartburn reduce stomach acid. Acid isn't always a bad thing. A car battery can't function without acid. Your digestive system can't either. The stomach acid breaks down foods and releases essential nutrients. Furthermore, reducing stomach acid also leaves the stomach at the mercy of germs and bacteria that cause food poisoning and other maladies.

Laboratory studies with rats have demonstrated that antioxidants, from fresh fruits and vegetables, do more to heal acid reflux disease than prescription medications!

These tips might help relieve the discomfort and potentially dangerous disease state that can be caused by acid reflux.

Eating

- Eat smaller amounts, more often, to avoid pressure in the abdomen.
- Avoid offending foods: fried foods, soft drinks, chocolate, coffee and alcohol.
- Change your diet to include 75% raw foods (fruits, vegetable and whole grains).
- For gentle relief, wash a raw potato. Put it in a juicer or blender. Mix with equal parts water and drink as needed.
- At the first sign of trouble, drink a large glass of water.

Body Mechanics

- Use gravity to help relieve chronic nighttime heartburn. Do not lie down flat for at least 3 hours after meals. Elevate the head of the bed with a four inch block.
- When sleeping, lie on your left side. This keeps the bulk of the stomach lower than its upper opening.

Helpful Supplements

- Enhance impaired digestion with live food enzymes
- Consider taking DGL or aloe vera to heal the lining of the G.I. tract.
- Some people find relief from betaine HCL or apple cider vinegar, 1 tablespoon before meals, for more complete digestion and less delay in emptying the stomach (delay can cause allergic reactions).
- Use natural enzymes for proper digestion. Take before meals. Pancreatin is best.

Avoid

- Avoid antacids! An overly acidic stomach does not cause heartburn. Maalox, Rolaids, Mylanta and other antacids contain aluminum; Tums, and others, contain calcium. Both aluminum and calcium can rebound (increase) acidity, causing further discomfort and need for more antacids. Aluminum is linked to Alzheimer's Disease. Baking soda can cause sodium overload over time.
- Avoid prescription medications such as Pepcid AC, Prilosec, Tagamet, Zantac, *et. al.* They block normal body processes, impair proper digestion of food and impede mineral absorption. Long-term use of these medications can damage the stomach lining and increase risk of benign and cancerous tumors.
- Avoid stress and anger.
- Avoid estrogen, e.g. birth control pills, menopause treatment. It can cause the lower muscles of the esophagus to weaken.
- Avoid smoking; it aggravates heartburn.

16

High Blood Pressure Pointers

You hear a lot about high blood pressure these days. Problem is, you may not have heard whether you have it or not. That's because high blood pressure goes about its destructive business in a very quiet manner. You can have it and not even suspect it.

So, first things first. If you haven't had your blood pressure checked recently, get it checked. Chances are, your county health department, church, local hospital or neighborhood medical clinic offers free blood pressure screening. Or, call your doctor's office. You wouldn't take a road trip if you weren't sure about your tire pressure. Your journey to optimal health requires just as much attention. Check your blood pressure!

What Is High Blood Pressure?

Blood pressure is the pressure exerted by your blood on the walls of your blood vessels. Blood pressure values are universally stated in millimeters of mercury (mmHg). The systolic pressure is pressure in your arteries during the peak of your cardiac cycle; diastolic pressure measures the pressure at the resting phase of the cardiac cycle.

Nerve impulses cause your arteries to dilate (become larger) or contract (become smaller). When these vessels are wide open, blood flows easily. When they narrow, it's harder for the blood to flow and the pressure inside them increases. This causes the heart and arteries to work harder and eventually damages them. Other organs, like the kidney, may become strained, too. The higher your blood pressure and the longer it goes untreated, the more you damage your heart, arteries and kidneys.

What Causes High Blood Pressure?

In about 90% of people with high blood pressure, no actual cause is found. However, high blood pressure is more common in African Americans, middle-aged and elderly people, obese people, heavy drinkers and women taking birth control pills. Some families seem predisposed to high blood pressure, but many with such a family history never get it. People with certain chronic diseases, including diabetes, gout and kidney disease, are more likely to have high blood pressure.

Your blood pressure is determined by four main factors:
- Your heart rate, how fast your heart pumps.
- Your blood volume, how much blood you have in your body.
- The resistance of your blood vessels. The higher the

resistance, the higher your blood pressure.
* Viscosity, how thick your blood is.

People with high blood pressure are often warned to decrease salt intake. Salt may increase your blood volume. People with high cholesterol are warned to lower it as high cholesterol levels can cause the build up of plaque in the arteries and increase their resistance. Blood thinners encourage blood to flow more quickly through the vessels.

What Does High Blood Pressure Cause?

While most people with high blood pressure don't know what caused it, we do know what high blood pressure causes. High blood pressure puts you at risk for strokes, heart attacks, heart failure, arterial aneurysms, and is the second leading cause of kidney failure in people with diabetes.

Take the Pressure Off

Making lifestyle changes can help you keep your blood pressure at healthy levels.
* **Reduce the amounts of fatty foods you eat**. Try to eliminate saturated fats. They are the worst culprits! All animal fats, fats found in meat, poultry and dairy products are saturated. Processed and fast foods also have saturated fats. Even vegetable oils can be saturated, for example, palm, palm kernel and coconut oils are saturated fats. All vegetable oils become saturated when they undergo a food processing technique called hydrogenation. Read the label—if the product contains hydrogenated vegetable oil, it contains unhealthy, saturated fats.
* **Quit smoking. Drink less alcohol.** Both can contribute to high blood pressure as well as heart attack and stroke.
* **Build your diet around whole, organic foods**, eaten raw or cooked from scratch. Recent studies confirm that a

fiber-rich diet reduces the occurrence of clogged arteries and hence, high blood pressure. You'll find fiber in fresh fruits, vegetables, legumes (beans) and whole grains.

Perhaps you believe it would be easier to just take medications to control high blood pressure. You probably know many people who do. While medications do have their time and place, they also have their side effects. If you can maintain healthy blood pressure without drugs, you won't have to worry about potentially dangerous side effects.

Drug Dangers

Diuretics (water pills) reduce blood volume by removing excess salt and water from the body
- Generic & corresponding Brands: Hydrochlorothiazide, Carozine, Diaqua, Esidrix, HydroDuiril, Microzide, Oretic
- Known side effects: Dizziness, lack of urination, muscle weakness and cramping, irregular heartbeat.

Vasodilators improve blood flow by relaxing muscles in blood vessel walls to open them up.
- Generic & corresponding Brands: guanabenz (Wytensin), dozazosin (Carduara), guanfacine (Tenex), guanethidine (Ismelin), methyldopa (Aldomet), prazosin (Minipress), terazosin (Hytrin), reserpine (Diupres), hydralazine (Apresoline), minoxidil (Loniten)
- Known side effects: Rapid heartbeat, headache, fluid retention, impotence, gastrointestinal problems (hydralazine), hair growth (monoxidil)

Alpha Blockers improve blood flow by reducing nerve impulses to blood vessel muscles.
- Generic & Corresponding Brands: doxazosin, (Carduara)

clonidine, prazosin, (Minipress), guanfacine (Tenex)
- Known side effects: Rapid heartbeat, headache, fluid retention, impotence, gastrointestinal problems, nightmares, numbness or tingling in hands and nausea.

17

IBS: A Personal and Social Nightmare

Irritable Bowel Syndrome (IBS) is a combination of symptoms that lead to tenderness, throbbing and agonizing pain accompanied by bloating, embarrassing flatulence and either incontinent diarrhea or obstructive constipation. Other symptoms include:
- Acid-reflux
- Groin pain and contractions
- Stomach cramping and pain
- Exhaustion
- Lower back pain
- Shooting pain in your hips and legs
- Inability to mentally focus
- Anxiety attacks
- Changes in heart rate and light headedness
- Constant weight gain

These symptoms arise when your digestion system fails to completely digest your food.

Eight of ten IBS patients report it as a progressive condition that can disable them within only a few years from the point of experiencing the first symptom.

Over the past ten years, Irritable Bowel Syndrome (IBS) has become the most widespread digestive ailment in the United States. Traditional medicine has no diagnosis for it, so it's labeled as a syndrome. Most physicians do not know how to remedy IBS; too often medical treatments are inadequate and ineffective.

If you suffer irritable bowel syndrome (IBS) or other digestive upsets, you may be spending a lot of money on over-the-counter and prescription remedies to treat your painful symptoms. The trouble is, symptoms are only a signal—a way your body communicates that something is not right. Taking a Tums or popping a Zelnorm may make you feel better temporarily, but such measures do not address the root cause of the upset. In fact, masking symptoms—and ignoring what your body is trying to tell you--can cause your health problems to get worse.

Your intestines take charge of a miraculously interactive process that releases and absorbs nutrients from the foods you eat, nutrients needed for healthy living. A phenomenal relationship between the brain and the gut takes place on a molecular level as neuropeptides and serotonins guide absorption of the released nutrients traveling through the intestines.

Without well-absorbed nutrients, none of the body's systems can enjoy optimum health. When the bowel is out of balance, it belches, burns, cramps, holds in or explodes.

Often, prescribed antispasmodic drugs (e.g. Lomotil) and diarrhea remedies (e.g. Immodium) slow intestinal function, causing serious side effects as well as dependency. Steroid drugs, cholesterol-lowering drugs and **sulfasalazines (Azulfidise, prescribed for ulcerative colitis), can make matters worse as they can interfere with absorption in the intestines.** Addictive tranquilizers and antidepressants can be equally dangerous.

IBS: The Cause

Many speculations have been made on the causes of IBS: genetics, infection, immune disorders, stress and diet. IBS is much more common in societies with a "Western" diet, like that eaten in the US; IBS virtually does not exist in societies where food is eaten fresh and prepared from scratch without additives and preservatives. Keeping that in mind, the first way to attack IBS is to defend your digestive system from the foods that are upsetting it.

If you experience the symptoms of IBS, you can start by avoiding:

- Sugar
- Caffeine
- Alcohol
- Fatty Foods
- Carbonated beverages
- Processed Foods

Food allergies can also trigger IBS symptoms. Common trigger foods include:

- Cow's milk
- Wheat
- Yeast
- Eggs
- Soy
- Corn
- Chocolate
- Citrus fruits.

Prescription medicines, lack of sleep and stress can also lead to IBS.

Finding Relief

Because a poor diet causes IBS, a good diet can help heal it. Eat healthy foods. A diet that includes plenty of fresh fruits, vegetables and whole grains is easier to digest. Consume natural, organic foods, raw or prepared from scratch. In fact, live, uncooked food is better when possible.

Meat and dairy products may contribute to upset. Eat slowly, while you're relaxed and chew every bite well. Digestion starts in the mouth—your saliva has enzymes that start the process!

Processed, fast food and refined foods contain large amounts of fat, sugar and irritating additives. The time you save in the fast food line may be wasted later as you are sidelined by pain and extra time in the bathroom.

To decrease inflammation, take one tablespoon of flaxseed oil every day. You can use this as a salad dressing or stirred into hot cereals or juice. Aloe vera can help heal your irritated intestinal walls. A good multi-vitamin/mineral supplement can help your body recover from months of not absorbing your food well. To rebalance your digestive system, include a fiber supplement, acidophilus and a good enzyme formula.

As stress is also a factor contributing to IBS, manage it with exercise, relaxation and plenty of sleep. Schedule a therapeutic massage, take a walk outdoors every day or wind down your night with a nice hot soak in the tub.

18
Insulin Resistance, Diabetes and Syndrome X

The American Obesity Association states that 127 million (64.5%) of U.S. adults are overweight and 60 million (30.5%) are obese. Diabetes among Americans is practically pandemic. Heart disease, with help from its cohorts, high blood pressure and high cholesterol, is the number one killer. Studies have found a common denominator among all of these conditions: insulin resistance.

What is Insulin Resistance?

A hormone secreted by the pancreas, insulin unlocks cells so they can convert glucose into energy. When insulin resistance occurs, the cells stay locked tight and the glucose builds up in the blood, causing high blood sugar. As a result, the pancreas manufactures more insulin. The excess insulin in the blood causes the liver to manufacture excess cholesterol.

In severe cases of insulin resistance, the cells fail to unlock—no matter how much insulin the pancreas secretes. Over time, the pancreas' ability to release insulin declines and blood sugar levels rise. The ultimate result? Type 2 diabetes. However, before people even suspect insulin resistance, they may find maintaining a healthy weight is difficult or impossible.

What Are the Signs of Insulin Resistance?

- Excess fat around the waist and buttocks.
- Inability to lose weight and maintain weight loss.
- Lack of energy, especially in the afternoon and after meals.
- Lack of concentration and mental fatigue.

Fueling Weight Gain, Foiling Weight Loss

During digestion, the body turns carbohydrates—bread, pasta, rice and sweets—into glucose (sugar). The normal American diet includes many highly processed carbohydrates and refined sugars; the pancreas must work overtime to manufacture enough insulin to handle all the glucose. When the cells say "enough is enough" and become insulin resistant, the body begins to store the excess blood sugar as fat. When cells develop insulin resistance, the body goes into hibernation mode--always tired and always hungry.

Insulin resistance causes the body to store more fat while preventing the body from burning fat as energy (decreased metabolism). Insulin resistance is more than a trait found in overweight and obese people—it may well be the root cause of their weight problem.

People following popular low-fat diets may encounter an additional challenge to weight loss. In an online report, the

Stanford University School of Medicine noted, "Research indicates that low fat diets may aggravate the effect of insulin resistance on blood lipids."

Syndrome X: The Disease Link

The link of insulin resistance to life-threatening diseases has turned it into a billion-dollar watchword in medical circles. Syndrome X is the term used for a cluster of risk factors for heart disease: hypertriglyceridemia (high blood lipid), low HDL-cholesterol, hyperinsulinemia (high blood insulin), hyperglycemia (high blood glucose) and hypertension (high blood pressure). All these risk factors have been linked to insulin resistance.

One in four of the 60 million Americans diagnosed with insulin resistance will develop type 2 diabetes. Insulin resistance also increases risk of stroke and blood lipid imbalances that lead to atherosclerosis. The excess insulin in the blood triggers the liver to manufacture more cholesterol

A diagnosis of insulin resistance is usually not made until people are diagnosed with one of the above diseases. Insulin resistance can be treated with two prescription drugs: pioglitazone and glimepirid. As with many pharmaceuticals, their use can result in a barrage of side effects, including weight gain.

Reversing Insulin Resistance

Reversing insulin resistance starts with practical advice. Be active. Exercise on a regular basis. Count calories. And, eat well—preferably a diet including:

- Five to nine servings of fruits and vegetables (the fresher the better)
- Five to eight ounces of protein
- Two to five servings of 100% whole grains (bread, pasta, rice)
- Two to three servings of dairy
- Two to three tablespoons of healthy fats.

- A good, daily multiple vitamin containing chromium and vanadium, two vital blood-sugar regulators.

Organic foods are always preferable. So is cooking from scratch—additives used in processed foods, like high fructose corn syrup, also build hard-to-lose belly fat.

Don't waste your time on fad diets. Don't wait for the diagnosis of disease. Work with your body naturally. Eat good foods. Exercise regularly.

19

Menopause and Native American Herbal Remedies

Long before Europeans colonized the Americas, Native Americans were wisely using the root of black cohosh to treat menstrual difficulties, ease menopausal symptoms and aid childbirth. The Delaware combined black cohosh with other herbs as tonic for female members of the tribe. The Iroquois brewed a strong tea from the root. They also used it as a footbath and to treat rheumatism. Likewise, the Cherokee used the roots to treat many different female conditions.

University of Michigan-Dearborn Native American Ethnobotany Database notes that the Algonkian, Micmac and Penobscot peoples also relied on the medicinal properties of black cohosh.

American herbalists learned about the efficacy of black cohosh from their Native American neighbors. Its importance as a medicinal herb was first recorded in 1801. From 1820 to 1926, black cohosh root was listed as an official drug of the

United States Pharmacopoeia. Throughout the 1800s, white physicians routinely prescribed it to their patients. Black cohosh was sometimes called by different names: black snakeroot and macrotys. Today, black cohosh goes by the scientific names Actaea racemosa and Cimicifuga racemosa, and is also referred to as Black Baneberry.

An Herbal Renaissance

It has taken centuries for mainstream America to recognize the wisdom and beauty found in the beliefs and practices of our Native American neighbors. Now, many of us have come to respect their stewardship of the land and their reverence for animal life. We are also learning the efficacy of their healing practices, including the use of herbs.

The physician that introduced echinacea to the white medical community in the mid 1800s, Dr. John King, told his obstetrics students that black cohosh was his favorite remedy. He used it in his own practice and wrote that is was his primary treatment "in abnormal conditions of the principal organs of reproduction in the female." King's words piqued the attention of the medical community in Germany, where black cohosh has remained a commonly prescribed remedy even today.

In modern times, the American medical community looked to Germany for modern documented experience with this useful traditional American Indian remedy. As noted in Part 1, black cohosh has remained a popular remedy for menopausal symptoms there for the past 150 years.

By 1962, 14 clinical studies involving more than 1,500 participants had been published on the use of black cohosh in the treatment of pre-menopausal and menopausal symptoms. It was proven to reduce the severity and duration of hot flashes, relieve night sweats and improve depressive moods. Studies in the 80s and 90s not only confirmed these conclusions, but also showed black cohosh to be a safe, effective alternative to estrogen replacement therapy, a therapy that puts women at substantial risk for many deadly and dangerous side effects.

What Causes Menopausal Symptoms?

Declining estrogen levels are at the heart of menopausal symptoms. However, today's lifestyle can make those symptoms worse. Our diets often consist of highly processed foods; we breathe polluted air and drink fluoridated or chlorinated water. Harried schedules and information overload drive up our stress levels and we often do not take time to enjoy exercise, fresh air and sunshine.

What causes hot flashes? Instability in your small blood arteries and capillaries leads them to dilate. What causes the blues? Estrogens are psychoactive hormones; their changing levels may cause you to feel depressed, anxious or experience mood swings. You may feel a profound sense of loss as you lose your fertility. What causes vaginal dryness and loss of libido? Less estrogen can mean lower libido. When your body ceases to create natural lubrication, sex may be uncomfortable or even painful. As estrogen decreases, your skin may become drier and bruise easily. You may have problems with incontinence. Don't be alarmed. The diet suggestions below, along with an herbal supplement that includes black cohosh can help see you through.

Include plant estrogens in your diet: organic soy products and tofu, linseeds, chickpeas, lentils and mung beans.

- Reduce your sugar and junk foods.
- Monitor your salt intake.
- Avoid spicy food, hot drinks and alcohol that can aggravate hot flashes.
- Limit red meat to one or two portions each week.
- Use safflower, sunflower, olive, sesame and rapeseed oils instead of animal fats.
- Include foods high in calcium and magnesium: milk, leafy green vegetables, unsalted nuts and seeds, whole grains

and sardines.
- Consume natural, organic foods: raw or prepared from scratch. Include fresh fruits, vegetables and whole grains.
- Drink eight to twelve glasses of pure water daily.

20
Osteoporosis: No Bones about It!

A progressive disorder, osteoporosis causes your bones to become weaker and weaker, leading to changes in posture and putting you at risk for bone fractures and life-changing complications.

If you've noticed that you've gradually lost your former height, your shoulders have become more rounded or you have general aches and pains throughout your body, you may be a victim of osteoporosis.

To prevent and control osteoporosis, you should take a three-prong attack: exercise, nutrition and sunshine.

Exercise

Consistent, moderate, weight bearing exercise not only decreases bone loss, it also increases bone mass. When you are inactive, calcium, the bone building mineral, leeches out of your system in urine and stool. The following forms of exercise benefit people at risk for or diagnosed with osteoporosis.

Strength training. Free weights, weight machines, resistance bands or water exercises strengthen the muscles and bones in your arms and upper spine; slows mineral loss from bones; and maintains flexibility in your spine.

Weight-bearing aerobic exercise. Walking, dancing, low-impact aerobics and gardening, work directly on the bones in your legs, hips and lower spine to slow mineral loss. They also reduce your risk of heart disease.

Flexibility exercises. By increasing joint mobility, you improve posture. Chest and shoulder stretches may be helpful, as may prone push-ups. Perform stretches after your muscles are warmed up, at the end of your exercise session.

Movements to avoid if you have osteoporosis:

- High-impact exercises, such as jumping, running or jogging. These can lead to fractures in weakened bones.
- Exercises in which you bend forward and twist your waist, such as touching your toes, doing sit-ups or using a rowing machine. These compress the bones in your spine. Other activities requiring these actions are golf, tennis, bowling and some yoga poses.

Nutrition

Calcium deficiency and bone loss are often symptoms of a larger dietary problem. Good sources of calcium include broccoli, dark leafy greens, kelp, oats, sesame seeds, soybeans and wheat germ.

Eat a whole foods diet based on fresh fruits and vegetables and 100% whole grains. Be sure to include fresh garlic and onions as you cook healthy dinners from scratch. These both contain sulfur, another mineral important for strong bones.

Organic soy products can also slow bone loss. (Beware: soybeans that are not certified organic may be genetically modified and dangerous for your overall health.

Take a high quality, natural multi vitamin/mineral formula which contains vitamins: C, D, E, K, B6 and B12 and minerals: calcium-magnesium, boron, zinc, copper, silicon, manganese and chromium. Chromium improves bone density and insulin efficiency. Avoid synthetic vitamins and poorly vitalized forms of calcium such as calcium carbonate.

Instead of exposing yourself to the risks of prescription

bone-loss drugs or dangerous hormone replacement therapy, supplement with DHEA, a natural alternative to hormone replacement.

What to Avoid:

- Excess protein, especially from meat and dairy products.
- Sugar. Sugar promotes calcium loss as do coffee (caffeine), alcohol and smoking.
- Carbonated beverages (soda pop). These contain phosphates, which leech calcium and other bone-friendly minerals from your system into your urine.

Last but not least . . . get out in the fresh air and enjoy the sunshine whenever you can. Exposure to sunlight, even just 15 minutes on the face, arms and hands, helps your body build bones with your calcium stores.

21
Pulse Testing for Food Allergies

Dr. Don suggests using the Pulse Test to quickly identify foods that cause allergic reactions. Test only one food a day!

1. Before getting out of bed in the morning, take your resting pulse. Using your index finger on the thumb side of your other wrist, count the number of beats you feel in one minute. Write this number down.

2. Eat the food you want to test. Only eat one food or you won't know which caused the reaction.

3. Remain in a rested position. After ten minutes, take your pulse again. Record.

4. Remain in a rested position. After an additional ten minutes, take your pulse again. Record.

Compare your first pulse rate with the following two. If you see an increase of ten or more beats per minute, chances are you have identified a food that causes you to have an allergic reaction. Eliminate this identified food from your diet.

22

Sinus Problems: A Real Drain!

An inflammation of the mucous membranes in the nasal sinuses, sinusitis can be cause by food allergies, infection or other factors that weaken the immune system. Symptoms include facial pain or tenderness, headache, earache, toothache, low-grade fever or difficulty breathing through your nose.

When you have a sinus problem, two goals should be kept in mind:
1. Preventing the sinus membranes from further swelling, and
2. Assisting the body in draining the mucous.

To accomplish these goals, follow the suggestions below:

Prevent swelling
- Identify food allergies and eliminate allergic foods from your diet. The most common culprits are milk, wheat,

yeast, eggs, corn, citrus fruits and peanut butter. To identify which foods cause you problems, use an elimination diet or pulse testing.
- Eat a 75% raw diet consisting of fruits, vegetables and whole grains.
- Upgrade your nutrition with a high quality multivitamin/ mineral formula that includes plenty of antioxidants, Vitamins A , C and E and selenium.
- Eliminate sugar (do not substitute artificial sweeteners. A moderate amount of Stevia maybe tolerated.)

Promote drainage
- Breathe steam under a towel tent for ten minutes, several times a day. You can add eucalyptus or menthol to increase effectiveness.
- Apply a warm towel to your sinus area for 20 minute. Then, lay down with your head lower than the rest of your body to help your sinuses drain.
- Irrigate your sinuses with a mixture of 1 cup warm water, ½ tsp. salt and a pinch of baking soda. Syringe into your nostrils and gently blow your nose.
- Use the herb Ma Huang to relieve congestion and swelling. In difficult cases, use goldenseal, a natural anti-infective and immune stimulator, and bromelain to help break up the mucous.
- Replace healthy bacterial flora with L. Acidophilus.

Avoid antibiotics, antihistamines and nose sprays
If you suspect infection, use colloidal silver, garlic, pycnogenols and aloe vera juice to boost your immune system. Antihistamines and nose sprays interfere with normal sinus drainage.

23

Thyroid Health: Common Sense Tips

When your thyroid is not functioning at full speed, your whole health suffers. Thyroid problems are frequently related to food allergies. So, your first step is to identify offending foods through an elimination diet or pulse testing. (See Regimen #20, Pulse Testing.)

Next, rule out any other contributing factors. Heavy metal poisoning, parasites, hypoglycemia and yeast syndrome can all impact thyroid health.

Diet
- Eat 4 to 5 smaller meals every day.
- Drink 8 to 12 glasses of pure filtered water daily.
- Begin with a 50% raw food diet based on fruits, vegetables and 100% whole grains.
- Eat a variety of whole grains; include millet and brown rice.
- For protein, eat raw nuts, seeds and cold water fish (e.g. salmon).
- Sprout your own lentils or alfalfa seeds, or purchase fresh organic sprouts to add to salads and sandwiches.
- Avoid animal products (i.e., meat and dairy).
- Avoid nightshade vegetables: potatoes, tomatoes, peppers, eggplant and tobacco.
- Abstain from sugar, coffee (caffeine) and alcohol.
- Supplement your diet with a high quality multivitamin and mineral formula that includes natural antioxidants and glandulars (adrenal and liver).
- Supplement with chlorophyll tablet or "green" drinks.

Daily Habits

- Establish a consistent exercise routine that includes stretching and light to moderate exercise.
- Sleep at least eight hours every night.
- Cleanse your colon with psylium or casgara sagrada herbs.
- Alternate hot/cold showers to stimulate circulation.

24

What Happens when I Drink Caffeine? When I Drink Pop? When I Drink Cows' Milk? When I Drink Alcohol?

You've heard the old cliché, "You are what you eat." Well, you are what you drink, too. It has been only in the past few decades that soda pop and sugary juice drinks have become beverage staples, served with every meal. Today, most grocery store milk is laced with hormones and antibiotics. And, while millions depend on coffee to get started or alcohol to unwind, have they really considered what this dependence is doing to their health?

Coffee? Decaf?

Caffeine gives you a kick, but also kicks your kidneys into distress. Do you have chronic back pain? Knee pain? Try cutting caffeine and see what happens. Coffee also causes excess loss of calcium in the urine and creates the potential for cadmium toxicity. Cadmium replaces the body's zinc stores, a health issue since zinc is one of the most important minerals for a strong immune system and proper T-cells. Cadmium also promotes cancerous changes in the cells of the body.

Decaffeinated coffee still contains the cadmium and other chemicals used in processing, which make it even more toxic.

Try safer, natural alternatives for energy and clearer, more focused thinking, such as: Ginkgo, Yerba Maté, Biloba and Ginseng!

Soft Drinks?

Soft drinks are hard on your body. Soft drinks are made with excess sugar and phosphates; both cause calcium loss in urine. Excess dietary sugar also turns into fat and depletes the body of B vitamins, especially B_1 (thiamin). Low B_1 can cause mood changes and behavior disorders. Sugar also directly suppresses the immune system by lowering white blood cell activity.

Soft drinks lower your pH, acidifying the body and promoting aging and free radical damage. It takes more than 20 glasses of pure water to undo the affects of one soft drink.

Diet Soft Drinks?

NutraSweet and other artificial sweeteners are highly toxic. NutraSweet (Aspartame) breaks down in the body into poisonous methanol and cancer-causing formaldehyde. Diet products containing NutraSweet can cause dozens of symptoms including headache, fatigue, irritability, depression, seizures, craving for sweets and more. Forget about losing any extra pounds; this artificial sweetener actually causes weight gain.

Cow's Milk?

If you are a baby cow, milk is the drink for you. If not, you may have problems with milk's very high protein and fat content. Milk causes calcium loss in urine, provokes allergies and can cause any number of symptoms. Dairy farmers routinely feed their cows hormones and antibiotics. Antibiotic content can destroy normal bacteria in your G.I. track. Growth hormones in milk can promote tumor growth and early puberty. Milk can also contain parasites. If you must drink milk, buy organic. Organic rice or soymilk makes a great substitute.

Don't kids need cows' milk? As a doctor and father of four, I'd rather see you give your kids rice milk or soymilk instead. Keep in mind God designed cows' milk for *calves*. It's astonishingly high in protein and fat, and though it's billed as a great source of calcium, it actually causes calcium depletion. The extremely high protein content of cows' milk causes the kidneys to lose calcium in the urine. So even though cows' milk contains a large amount of calcium, drinking it actually results in a net *loss* of calcium from your body.

Cows' milk also provokes allergies (look at all the lactose intolerance these days) and contains antibiotics that destroy good bacteria in the gastrointestinal tract. It contains growth hormones that can promote tumor growth. When it's homogenized in processing, then it gets really scary. Homogenization and pasteurization turn milk into a manmade food containing more health liabilities than assets. Cow's milk is best left to baby cows.

Alcohol?

Alcohol is a poison that directly damages the brain, liver, pancreas and small intestine. The danger of killing brain cells is obvious. In the liver, fatty accumulations can lead to hepatitis, cirrhosis and eventually death. Damage to the pancreas can lead to diabetes.

Effects on the small intestine lead to poor absorption of all nutrients, especially the fat-soluble vitamins (A, D, E and K), the B vitamins, folic acid and vitamin C. This is particularly disturbing because many of these protect the body from free radical damage, which promotes aging and all diseases associated with aging (including heart diseases, cancer and arthritis). Alcohol can increase free radical formation making it a double-edged sword that speeds aging. It also directly suppresses the immune system and depletes the body of zinc (a major immune stimulating mineral).

Five leading causes of death are associated with the use of alcohol:

1. Car Accidents
2. Cirrhosis of the Liver
3. Pneumonia
4. Suicide
5. Murder

Get Wet!

According to the Biblical story of creation, on the first day, God created water. Water is the basis for life on earth. It is also the basis for the life of your body. The healthy adult body is 65% water; the healthy brain, 75 to 80% water. It's easy to see why water is the beverage of choice. For optimum health, drink at least eight, eight-ounce glasses of pure, filtered or distilled water every day. Municipal water supplies add chemicals such as fluoride, which has been linked to bone cancer; and chlorine, which kills beneficial intestinal flora, is linked to cancers and can impair skin, hair and nail health.

Part of the mystique of those other beverages is the ritual. Drink your water in a stemmed glass, on ice or hot in your favorite mug (brewed as an herbal tea). Enjoy, give thanks and be healthy!

25

Yeast Infection: A Clear and Present Danger

What is Yeast?

Yeast (Candida Albicans) naturally lives in your healthy digestive system: the mouth, throat, intestines and genitourinary tract. It is a normal bowel flora that destroys harmful bacteria, not a parasite. When Candida overgrows, it shifts into a fungal form that invades the body. It then causes vaginal yeast infections, oral thrush infestations and, when the fungal rhizoids penetrate intestinal walls, leaky gut syndrome, a condition that allows toxins, undigested food, bacteria and yeast to enter the bloodstream.

Symptoms of Candida fungal infection include:

- Cravings for Sweets
- Overall Feeling of Poor Health
- Embarrassing rectal or vaginal itch
- Splotchy Skin or Rashes

If your body has indeed been overrun by Candida albicans, you may also experience:

- Lack of energy: sleepiness, fatigue and always feeling tired and/or insomnia.
- Pain: muscle aches, headache, painful joints or numbness.
- Mental fog: inability to focus, mood swings, depression, crying jags and irritability.
- Sinus pain, dizziness and sore throat
- Bad breath and body odor.

- Gastrointestinal problems: constipation, diarrhea, bloating, gas, irritable bowel syndrome, abdominal cramps
- Respiratory problems: coughing, wheezing or shortness of breath.
- Loss of libido.

If you have any of the following medical conditions, you may also be a victim of Candida fungal infection:

- PMS and Menstrual Irregularities
- Fibromyalgia and Chronic Fatigue Syndrome
- Sexual Dysfunction
- Asthma and Allergies
- Food Allergies
- Ear Infections
- Psoriasis and Athlete's Foot
- Urinary Tract Problems
- Multiple Sclerosis
- Migraines

Common Signs of Candida Overgrowth

When you hear the term yeast infection, two well-known manifestations of this condition may come to mind.

Oral thrush.

A yeast infection on your tongue and inside your cheeks, thrush results in creamy white lesions that may bleed slightly when you scrape them or brush your teeth. If left untreated, thrush can spread to the roof of your mouth, gums, tonsils and back of your throat. Thrush occurs more often in babies, toddlers, older adults and those with compromised immune systems.

Severe thrush can travel down the esophagus and into the stomach, causing painful swallowing or the sensation that something is stuck in your throat.

Home remedies include eating plain yogurt; applying a solution made of 1 tsp. baking soda or one tablespoon of vinegar dissolved in 8 ounces of water. Or break open a capsule of acidophilus and rub it on the lesions.

Vaginal Yeast Infections

You've no doubt encountered advertisements promoting various products to eliminate vaginal yeast infections. Vaginal yeast infection results in a thick white cottage cheese-like discharge that causes painful irritation, constant itching and pain during intercourse. Home remedies include: using plain, unsweetened yogurt or a gauze wrapped, peeled garlic clove as suppositories. Dress so as not to restrict airflow. Wear a skirt or loose fitting pants, no panties to bed and avoid tight jeans and panty hose.

If you find thrush or vaginal yeast infections are a recurrent theme in your life, most likely the yeast overgrowth is not limited to these areas of inflammation.

The Yeast Epidemic

Many modern healthcare and hygiene practices stimulate Candida fungal infection. One common culprit is antibiotics. Antibiotics kill the good bacteria in our bodies along with the harmful bacteria. These good bacteria balance the naturally occurring Candida in our systems. When the good bacteria are killed, Candida overgrows. Chemicals, chlorinated water, antibiotics used in farm animals and meat processing and even pesticides in the environment stimulate Candida overgrowth. Our sugary foods feed Candida and cause overgrowth, as well. Virtually everyone today is at risk for Candida fungal infection.

Other factors that raise your risk of Candida overgrowth include:
- Steroids

- Uncontrolled diabetes
- Hormonal changes: pregnancy, using birth control pills and menopause

Bubble baths, vaginal contraceptives, damp or tight-fitting clothing and feminine hygiene sprays and deodorants can also increase your susceptibility to yeast infection.

Are You at Risk for Candida Overgrowth?

Answer the following questions. If you respond "yes" to seven or more, you probably already have a Candida overgrowth issue.

1. Has your doctor routinely prescribed antibiotics for ear infections, acne, respiratory infections or other reasons?
2. Have you ever been on a course of prednisone, steroids or birth control pills?
3. Do you eat a lot of dairy products, poultry, beef or pork from animals raised on antibiotics?
4. Do you feel sick all over but your doctor doesn't know why?
5. Is it sometimes hard to stay focused because you feel "spacey"?
6. Do cigarette smoke, perfumes or home fragrances give you headaches?
7. Do you have irritable bowel syndrome or any of its symptoms: constipation, diarrhea, bloating, excess gas?
8. Do you crave sugar?
9. Do you suffer with PMS, menstrual irregularities, low libido or sexual dysfunction?
10. Do you routinely suffer with vaginitis, rectal itch or thrush?
11. Do you have light "splotches" on the skin of your arms or legs, have dry skin or easily irritated skin?

Dangers of Candida Overgrowth

When Candida transforms from yeast into dangerous fungi, it seeps toxins that block normal nutrient absorption. Candida rhizoids take deep root in your intestinal walls causing symptoms of Irritable Bowel Syndrome.

Eventually, rhizoids perforate the intestines, causing Leaky Gut Syndrome. When Candida toxins get into your bloodstream, Systemic Candida can invade all of your organs and tissue.

Untreated Candida can trigger bowel disorders, food intolerance, environmental sensitivities, allergies and asthma. Candida can set off autoimmune disorders, such as chronic fatigue syndrome and fibromyalgia, as your body begins attacking itself at the cellular level.

Overcoming Candida Overgrowth

Cut Sugar. Yeast is an organism, and like all living creatures, needs food to live and multiply. What feeds yeast? Sugar. Have you ever baked homemade bread? If so, you've watched what happens when you mix the baking yeast with warm liquid and sugar in a bowl—it grows and froths and, when mixed with the other ingredients, its continued growth causes the bread to expand and rise.

The average American eats 53 teaspoons of sugar a day. If you're serious about stopping Candida overgrowth in its tracks, cut sugar out of your diet. That doesn't only mean sugary soft drinks, cookies, candy and sweets. Sugar hides in most of today's processed foods. Read the labels and root out sugar from your diet. You'll not only starve the yeast, you'll enjoy other health benefits as well.

Eat healthy foods. Focus on God-made foods: fresh fruits and vegetables, nuts and seeds, unprocessed oils and limited quantities of antibiotic-free meat, fish and eggs. Drink eight to ten glasses of pure, filtered water every day. Avoid flavored waters. If these don't contain sugars, they do contain artificial sweeteners that can wreak even more havoc on your health. If desired, substitute unsweetened green tea for up to four of your water servings daily.

Eating organic, plain yogurt with active probiotic cultures can help reintroduce balance to your system.

Rule Out Food Triggers. To rule out food allergy culprits in your diet, avoid the following foods for two weeks. Then introduce them, one at a time, to see what ill effects they may have on you:

- Yeast (breads made with it)
- Food coloring and additives
- Milk and dairy products
- Processed and packaged foods
- Wheat, Oats, Rice
- Beef , pork, chicken and eggs
- Coffee, tea, fruit punch, rice
- Citrus fruits, corn , tomatoes, white potatoes
- Chocolate

Supplement Your Diet
- Choose a high quality brand recommended by your alternative health. **Probiotics, such as Acidophilus, are** the friendly bacteria that the Candida has overrun. These helpful microorganisms help maintain the health of your digestive tract.
- **Digestive enzymes can** help maintain a natural, healthy digestion and reduce the occurrence of Candida in the intestines.
- **Herbals that help** inhibit the growth of *Candida include usnea, spilanthes*, pau d'Arco, oregano, oil, black walnut,

grapefruit seed extract, garlic, beta carotene, and biotin.

- **Daily multivitamin** and mineral supplements help your body fight off Candida overgrowth. Ask for recommendations from your alternative health practitioner or trusted nutraceutical source.

Don Ver Hulst, M.D., received his B.S. in Zoology at the University of Michigan in 1978 and his M.D. from Wayne State University School of Medicine in 1982. After graduating from medical school, he realized that his continual fast-food diet and late-night study habits had taken a serious toll on him physically. The adage "Physician, heal thyself" took on a whole new meaning for him as he struggled with his stressful and demanding career. When he accepted Christ into his heart, though, he felt that every page of the Bible began speaking to him about God's promises of health and wellness for every believer. He began studying the divine health principles in God's Word from a physician's viewpoint, and what he found amazed him with its simplicity and practicality. Dr. Don's 10 Keys to Cure were the result.

Today, Dr. Don embraces the naturopathic philosophy of health and has dedicated his life to teaching the principles of preventive medicine. His mission is to share God's simple and effective biblical health plan with as many people as possible. Dr. Don lectures in schools, churches, and other organizations, as well as on television and radio programs across the country.

Dr. Don loves spending time at home with his wife, Susan, who has hosted a Christian radio program for the last 20 years and who enjoys supporting her husband's work in the health and nutrition field. Together they spend lots of quality time with their four children, Donnie, Aidon, Jaclyn, and Vivian, who range in age from 3 to 10 years old. Dr. Don also enjoys cooking natural foods and working on his music.